CONTEMPORIZING HYPNOTHERAPY

Books of Same Author

- सत्य अहिंसा के प्रयोगः दलाईलामा का तिब्बत से निष्कासन (2008)
- Experiments with Truth and Non-Violence: The Dalailama in Exile from Tibet (2007)
- Experiments with Truth and Non-Violence: China Challenged (Revised and Enlarged) (2013)
- Indian Handbook of Hypnotherapy Foundations and Strategies (4th Edition)(2016)
- Contemporizing Raj Yoga: Neuroscience and Practices (2017)
- Space Time Consciousness: Rationale of Paranormal (2021)
- The Real Life Story of Stem Cells(2021)
- Contemporizing Pragnya: A Holistic ReVision (2023)

About the Authors

Dr. Bhaskar Vyas (1937) Plastic Surgeon and **Dr. Rajni Vyas** (1937) Obstetrician and Gynaecologist have contributed to their respective fields with research innovations. Dr. R. Vyas has made a seminal contribution to unexplained reproductive failure with a success rate of 55 per cent with her research protocol. This is highest success rate. Dr. B. Vyas' seminal contribution is to derive several products from stem cells obtained from fat. They have numerous research papers published. They have published over a score of books. Concept Publishing Company has published their books on the topic of philosophy, psychology and physics viz. *Contemporizing Raj Yoga*, *Experiments with Truth and Non-violence—China Challenged* 3rd Edition, *Indian Handbook of Hypnotherapy* 4th Edition, *Space Time Consciousness—Rationale of the Paranormal*, *Contemporizing Pragnya*. This book is the latest addition to the 'Contemporizing' series. The authors proudly describe themselves as perennial students of philosophy, continually seeking to expand their understanding and contribute to the advancement of knowledge in their fields.

Contemporizing Hypnotherapy

A Treatise in New Age

Bhaskar Vyas
Rajni Vyas

Edited by
Vatsal Naik

CONCEPT PUBLISHING COMPANY PVT. LTD.
NEW DELHI - 110 059

ISBN: 978-93-5594-712-3

First Published 2024

Published and Printed by

Concept Since 1974

Concept Publishing Company Pvt. Ltd.
A/15-16, Commercial Block, Mohan Garden
New Delhi-110059 (India)
T: +91-11-41101460
E: publishing@conceptpub.com, *W*: www.conceptpub.com

Cataloging in Publication--Courtesy: D.K. Agencies (P) Ltd. <docinfo@dkagencies.com>

Vyas, Bhaskar, author.
Contemporizing hypnotherapy : a treatise in new age / Bhaskar Vyas, Rajni Vyas ; edited by Vatsal Naik.
pages cm
Includes bibliographical references and index.
ISBN 9789355947123

1. Hypnotism--Therapeutic use. 2. New Age movement. 3. Mind and body. 4. Spiritual life--Hinduism. I. Vyas, Rajni, author. II. Naik, Vatsal, editor. III. Title.

LCC RC495.V93 2024 | DDC 615.8512 23

Foreword

In the realm of human consciousness, where the mind and its potentialities hold sway, lies a vast landscape awaiting exploration and transformation. It is within this captivating realm that the ancient practice of hypnotherapy finds its roots, offering a gateway to the deepest recesses of the human psyche. In this book, the authors endeavour to bridge the gap between the teachings of the Milton Erickson and the present age, revitalizing and contemporizing them for modernity.

As Indian authors, they bring with them a unique perspective, intertwined with the rich tapestry of their cultural heritage. Drawing inspiration from revered figures such as Rohit Mehta, Kripa Thakur, and Rishikesh Jana, who initiated the Indian Society of Hypnosis, they acknowledge the invaluable contributions of their predecessors. Their wisdom and experiences have paved the way for the authors to embark on this transformative journey, as they explore the realms of hypnotherapy and its potential to heal and alleviate the burdens of the human condition.

Their exploration extends beyond the traditional boundaries of hypnotherapy, delving into the realms of spirituality and the insights gleaned from luminaries such as Sri Aurobindo. They are fascinated by Einstein's revelation in his letter to Hadamard, where he described the nature of his thought process, receiving visual and aural stimuli that guided him. Building upon this foundation, they explore the profound connection between hypnotherapy and the power of thought, seeking to unleash its therapeutic potential to unlock the gates of healing. This book has a novel description of the technique for rapid induction, innovation to design a matrix by devising an altogether new fabric by incorporating music, and creative ideas thus far not explored.

In their pursuit of understanding the intricate workings of the mind, they delve into the intriguing world of gene expression and subsequent melatonin expression in hypnotic states and meditation.

The modern era, with its multitude of challenges and afflictions, calls for innovative approaches to healing and well-being. They explore the manifold uses of hypnotherapy in addressing modern-day maladies such as stress, anxiety, and trauma, drawing inspiration from the timeless wisdom of the *Bhagavad Gita*. They find parallels within its passages that mirror the concepts of indirect or direct hypnotherapy, using metaphors and archetypal symbols to penetrate the depths of the unconscious and effect profound change.

They explore the intricate interplay between hypnosis, hypnoanesthesia, unravelling the mysteries of age regression and its potential for healing deep-seated trauma.

In their exploration of the human mind, they are guided by the profound insights of *Icchashakti* and *Kriyashakti*, the creative and formative powers of thought, that have had profound implications as per Kashmir Shiva Agamas. With these potent tools at their disposal, they seek to empower the hypnotherapist, as they venture forth into the realm of hypnotherapy and its transformative potential.

The second part of this book presents a collection of hypnotherapeutic scripts, carefully crafted to address various ailments and afflictions that were successful. Drawing from diverse belief systems, they employ suggestions and metaphors that resonate with religious individuals, while also providing archetypal symbols to those who may not subscribe to any particular faith.

The book exhorts the therapist to innovate, to delve deep. May this work serve as a guiding light, illuminating the path to self-discovery and offering solace to those who look for the transformative potential of hypnotherapy.

This treatise heralds a new dawn for hypnotherapists to innovate and research.

Prof. Bimla Parimu

Preface

"Contemporizing Hypnotherapy: A Treatise in New Age" is a culmination of profound insights, extensive research, and invaluable experiences garnered by Dr. Rajni Vyas and Dr. Bhaskar Vyas in the field of hypnotherapy. This collaborative effort stems from a deep-rooted passion for exploring the intersections of ancient wisdom and modern therapeutic practices.

Our journey into the realm of hypnotherapy took an enlightening turn with the guidance of Kripa Thakur, whose teachings transcended mere instruction to delve into the realms of archetypal symbols and the rich tapestry of Indian heritage. It was under his mentorship that the seeds of the New Age concept were sown within us, prompting a fervent exploration of its relevance within the context of hypnotherapy. New Age has been heralded since the 1970s following the passing of Milton Erickson. Now, the term "New Age" is familiar to various disciplines for its inclusion of a spiritual dimension.

Dr. Rajni Vyas, with her profound understanding of the term "New Age", spearheaded a discourse that aimed to infuse this ethos into the very fabric of our therapeutic endeavours. Through tireless dedication to practice, research, and innovation, she paved the way for groundbreaking discoveries that continue to shape the landscape of hypnotherapy in India today.

In an era characterized by rapid change and evolving societal paradigms, the need to contemporize hypnotherapy is more pressing than ever before. As the demand for holistic and spiritually grounded approaches to healing surges, it becomes imperative for hypnotherapists to adapt and expand their skill sets accordingly.

This book serves as a guide for hypnotherapists seeking to navigate the complexities of the New Age landscape. With a meticulous blend of theory, practical techniques, and insightful strategies, it aims to empower practitioners with the tools necessary to meet the diverse needs and aspirations of individuals in the modern world.

As you embark on this transformative journey through the pages of Contemporizing Hypnotherapy, may you find inspiration, wisdom, and practical guidance to enhance your practice and make a meaningful difference in the lives of those you serve.

Bhaskar Vyas
Rajni Vyas

Contents

1

Introduction

We, the authors of the book 'Contemporizing Hypnotherapy' in year 2024, like to describe ourselves as children walking on the seashore and wondering, while gathering fables at the vast expanse of the seashore. Our state of mind is like to be wondering at the vast expanse, not only of the seashore but eternity of time, endless expanse of the space, and lost in the thought as to where did consciousness begin in the universe. Such a reflection, we have expressed through more than a score of books but a wonderful fable that works like a magic stone to help humanity and we add with emphasis that even animals.

Being scientifically inclined, we asked our friend, philosopher and guide, Dr. Anand Bhushan Khorana. He was an enlightened psychiatrist. He introduced for the first time to us the world of hypnosis. When asked, 'But how does hypnosis work?', he took us to a workshop at Ahmedabad where Dr. Rishikesh Jana, a physiologist was conducting a two day introductory workshop. Along with him there were Dr. Athavale and a gynaecologist, Dr. Modi. There being three medical doctors and we are being guided by a psychiatrist added to our faith in what we are seeing and experiencing.

Dr. Athavale demonstrated anaesthesia of half an arm all the way down to the fingertips. However, the proximal arm was having full sensation. This does not collate with anatomical description but that has happened! We decided on our return to Baroda to conduct such a workshop at Medical Association. All the three and additionally Dr. Khorana, to add emphasis on a sceptical audience, conducted a day long introductory workshop on hypnosis. Its utilization in therapy was left out to be pursued not only by the audience but by ourselves as well.

A phenomenon to be described as only to prove its validity with a demonstration that has occurred. However, we thought there might be a philosophical elucidation available. We asked Rohit Mehta, our mentor in philosophy. He guided us to read and revise both the volumes of 'Talks with Sri Aurobindo' and to our utter surprise, we found that Sri Aurobindo has also pondered what is hypnosis. Sri Aurobindo has said, "In other words, does the quality of a thing depend on the object or on the subject? Take, for instance, beauty. When we call someone or something beautiful, is it because the object itself is beautiful or the subject sees it as such—that is, does beauty depend only on the psychological state of the subject and have nothing to do with the object? But is this reaction confined to humanity or is it a common reaction of all living beings? Hypnotism is a supraphysical state, and the ordinary physical laws bringing about the ordinary reactions are not valid then. One shouldn't do these things except under guidance or in the presence of a Master."

Rohit Mehta further guided us to the use of metaphors that drive the point indirectly and yet, certainly. He explained that *Upanishads*[1] were written in story telling style when most students found the *Vedas*[2] as terse and direct, without further elucidation. The *Rishis*[3] of the yesteryears therefore took resort to storytelling through *Upanishads*. Each *Upanishad* is a story based on curiosity, extending to further expansion with questioning and delivering a message through a story.

Rohit Mehta was endowed with a vast repertoire from references from Sri Aurobindo as well as theosophical literature. He referred us to study what Sri Aurobindo has said about hypnotherapy (while hypnosis as a phenomenon was widely discussed by philosophers, its usage as a therapy was not even thought of. That is why Sri Aurobindo refers the phenomena as hypnotism. In contemporary times, all –isms have become –wasms. So only hypnotherapy should prevail.)

Sri Aurobindo has written in 'Life Divine' as follows, "From this nature of mental and sense knowledge as it is at present organised in us, it follows that there is no inevitable necessity in our existing limitations. They are the result of an evolution in which mind has accustomed itself to depend upon certain physiological functioning and their reactions as its normal means of entering into relation with the material universe. Therefore, although it is the rule that when we seek to become aware of the external world, we have to do so indirectly through the sense organs and can experience only so much of the truth about things and men as the senses convey to us, yet this rule is merely the regularity of a dominant habit. It is possible for the mind—and it would be natural for it, if it could be persuaded to liberate itself from its consent to the domination of matter,—to take direct cognisance of the objects of sense without the aid of the sense-organs. This is what happens in experiments of hypnosis and cognate psychological phenomena. Because our waking consciousness is determined and limited by the balance between mind and matter worked out by life in its evolution, this direct cognisance is usually impossible in our ordinary waking state and has therefore to be brought about by throwing the waking mind into a state of sleep which liberates the true or subliminal mind."

We see that in the phenomena of hypnosis not only can the hypnotised subject be successfully forbidden to feel the pain of a wound or puncture when in the abnormal state, but can be prevented with equal success from returning to his habitual reaction of suffering when he is awakened. The reason of this phenomenon is perfectly simple; it is because the hypnotiser suspends the habitual waking consciousness which is the slave of nervous habits and is able to appeal to the subliminal mental being in the depths, the inner mental being who is master."

It surprised us to read what Sri Aurobindo has written, which now we will term as 'Self Hypnosis'. Sri Aurobindo further writes under the caption of 'Delight of Existence' as, "But this freedom which is effected by hypnosis abnormally, rapidly, without true possession, by an alien will, may equally be won normally, gradually, with true possession, by one's own will so as to effect partially or completely a victory of the mental being over the habitual nervous reactions of the body."

This collateral sustenance by a profound philosopher that Sri Aurobindo was, confirmed our faith to take hypnosis to hypnotherapy. Today there are several different methods to treat various ailments of body and mind. The success rate may depend on the acceptance by the patient and the mastery of the hypnotherapist.

That is the rising of the consciousness out of the body. In hypnosis the subjects can know all their experiences.

Rohit Mehta drew our attention to Patanjali's *Yoga Sutra*. Patanjali, in the *Vibhutipada*[4] has described a spontaneous accrual of 8 *Siddhis*[5] of which *Vashita*[6], which translates as ability to hypnotize, is one. The meditative state has to be practiced for a number of years. In modern age of high speed, who has the time and patience to wait for 12 years or more? Meditation, when compared to a climbing staircase, may lead to self-realization and simply as a higher state of oneself while hypnotherapy is like climbing the topmost floor with a well-defined destination that can be even monitored by a therapist.

Rohit Mehta further enlightened the way by inaugurating Baroda Hypnosis Society where Dr. Udar, a pathologist and Dr. Ratubhai Parikh were the first office bearers.

Take this as a parody; take it really seriously: Fact of the matter is Hypnotherapy is a Science

This may sound to be a platitude for those who are learned and practicing hypnotherapy with demonstrable results. However, for those who find them novice to the field, it does come as a surprise. Any idea that is novel, fascinating, luminous, dazzling or may be even, bizarre,—like a girl in the magic box being cut into two and jumping alive as one—produces a specific response from the observer. That also is common sense: One gets dazed and at times aghast! Hypnotic processes and magical demonstrations both appear extraordinary and yet, there is no magic about it: and, both are based on certain psychodynamic processes that are just being discovered—though such phenomena are a part of our everyday life! Even noting certain details at a murder or terror scene and forgetting some is based on functioning of certain neurons and genes (!) at such times.

People mistakenly say; with the advent of quantum physics, Newtonian physics is outdated. They forget we are talking about an apple falling from a tree to the ground and the planets going round the solar system—even stock market functions as per the law of cause and effect! But did not Newton say that give me a long enough stick and make me stand in the solar system outside the earth and, I shall lift up the earth with my stick!" For those who take a cue from this and try to use the law of gravitation for pulling money out of stock market through self-hypnosis—thinking themselves to be great telepathic programmers of the markets forget the elementary principle that in gravitational pull mass is the important factor. The gravitational pull of greed can be like a black hole so that huge finance institutions across the world also get sucked shrunk and disappear. This is also hypnotic process as a science. So science is all about cause and effect, that cause causality to change the environment; results and variables, predictability and certainty. If physics and mathematics are such high precise sciences conforming to the principles of deductive logic, believe us when we say, hypnosis will also conform to those principles. Did not Sankaracharya say about the world being a mirage? *Brahmam satyam: jagat mithya!* If the entire world is a stage and we are but players in a drama, was Shakespeare not a great hypnotist to create such illusions that Romeo and Juliet still exist?

Some innocent genuinely nice people—to be innocent genuinely nice people is a hypnodrama being played most frequently by good, bad and ugly; all across the band—ask us: do you believe in ghosts? We refer them to Dr. Jekyll and Mr. Hyde. It is pathetic to see that Mr. Hyde is in most of us, most of the times—and some of us secretly love him too! And several expert psychiatric doctors; Jekyll cannot exorcise him. Yet it may take a fresher in Clinical Psychology who has just walked out of the hypnosis workshop, a few sessions with hypnosis that the pathological ego states gets fused into one forever.

Freshers will crack the psychodynamics of schizophrenics by just cataloguing the few years backwards of a young man to discover when was it that he was bit by a scorpion girl—*vishkanya*[7] to be precise—that left him beaten, battered and perceptually blind so as to have disorientation in time and space. Most high profile psychiatrists will revel in uncovering the schizophrenic gene and keep changing molecules after molecules for this young man. Yes, they are right in ridiculing psychoanalysis as the pursuit of lazy nineteenth century psychologists. Who has the time today to browse, read and mull over *Romeo and Juliet! All the world is a stage, and we the doctors are just the actors in the melodrama that is played about: let us do our role to prescribe and change from one molecule to another.* This may be an ordeal for most mentally wrecked, but even a naïve hypnotherapist age regresses empathetically to erase the traumatic memories by selective ablation of the past event. To follow up, even post hypnotic work so that the boy passes his final examination with distinction. That should remind us of the fact that John Nash winning a Nobel Prize is a real life story.

Yet, if some credit is to be given to quantum physics as some kind of hypnodrama, it tells us about every particle changing its action with presence of an observer. Einstein refused to believe that a mouse looking at the Universe does change it. He said, God does not play dice. Neil Bohr's reply was: Let God do his work and physicists their own. The hard core psychopharmocologists and psychiatrists would not believe that a tiny-mini clinical psychologist can look into the psychodynamics of a ravaged mind and, through the cyclic rotation of time dimension, can bring about a cure that would very soon be drugless.

The energy, which is unknowingly being provided by the consciousness of the observer in quantum physics, seems to be playing the same truant in the relationship between the subject and the therapist. The charisma of one influences reciprocally at times so great that one sees God when none exists. Poor hypnotherapist is trapped with the difficulty of studying the human behaviour which changes its route with presence of each different observer. There may be more interpretations of psychodynamics than the number of therapists and, none can be proved wrong! Knowing the real self, what lies deep within, what stirs up and stimulates within with every new experience; such questions are numerous! Like they say, knowing *Shiva* is enough for many, but for few it is the search of *Mahadev*, and for even fewer, it goes up to the search of *Mahakaal*.[8] As such, who would and who would not dare to discern the darkness which is lying deep within the realms of Unconsciousness? Once again, hypnotherapist will answer such questions most humbly that he is just a poor scientist: for him the success of such probing lies in restoring his subject to functionality.

Humans are the most trainable species, and we train our minds with everything that we see or listen or just experience. Why would the *Panch Tantra* tales be so effective in teaching a child about morals and discipline? Story telling being one of the oldest arts is enough to explain suggestibility and also to tell when someone is highly suggestible. We do not need to quote Milton Erickson—or for that matter us. We can easily find the references of ill/well effects of the daily television soap operas on the families following them. With the women having greater difficulty in finding peace and being content, and the men having trouble of searching the satisfaction with uncontrolled drive of ambition, we are talking about a society which is very high on indulgence. So, when a hypnotherapist cures a long history of infertility in just a few sessions, it is not miracle. It is a hundred per cent science that restores the *milleu interior* to normal natural pulsatility that someone out there programmed the female since the times of Eve.

Let us take a simpler case: What happens when a woman is humiliated for her good looks? Very simple, she develops twitching of face. It is wonderful to see hypnotherapeutic suggestions work and the women being rid of her six years long abysmal trouble in just sixty days!

After all this persuasion, if the reader is now convinced that hypnotherapy is indeed a science as much is surgery. Only a few centuries back, surgery was done by barbers. Ask Milton Erickson. He will carry on the tale till such times that you will end up convinced that any barber may become a surgeon but it requires a real creative genius to paint a Mona Lisa.

Milton Ericksons are not made: they happen as the flowering of the creative upsurge of a huge human potential. No hadron collider will ever produce a Leonardo da Vinci or a Milton Erickson!

A hypnotherapist is committed to help humanity at large. It is perfectly ethical for him to charge a reasonable fee since he has also to maintain a family and live himself. However, some people have been looted by lay hypnotists. This has given a bad name to the entire discipline. We have taken a vow that we will make Vadodara, India a Mecca of hypnotherapy but additionally add a spiritual dimension to that as well.

We got a seminal support from Prof. Bimla Parimu. She, with some consternation from her peers, decided to advocate with the University authorities and succeeded in introducing a diploma course in 2000 that goes on today as Diploma in Clinical and Applied Hypnosis.

When the support and response from the passing students increased, Bimla Parimu asked us to organize a conference. We got all round support from not only in India but even from United Kingdom. Ashwin Barot, an Ayurvedic physician, also registered with two United Kingdom citizens. One, a head of the department in anaesthesia while the other after graduating in modern medicine in UK, started practicing Ayurvedic medicine in Greece. Two psychiatrists came for the introductory workshop and made an issue with us as to why we have not made the workshop and conference widely circulated. Alok Prapanna, at the conference made a video presentation of how a burns patient, without resorting to any anaesthesia but simply under hypno-anaesthesia, would allow the insertion of a pin made of steel into the heads of four metacarpals and further allowed the taking of a skin graft. This all culminated into a wide publicity for acceptance of hypnotherapy as a respectable method.

We received invitations from across India. We organized several workshops at New Delhi, beginning with Vidyasagar Institute of Mental Health, Neuro and Allied Sciences—VIMHANS. Prof. Nathawat invited us to present with a keynote at Jaipur. Lata Hemchand, a delegate from NIMHANS sent his relation suffering from rheumatic gangrene extending from her shin to the top of the right ankle, about 8 inches by 4 inches ulcer. An orthopaedic surgeon advised amputation below knee. The patient's relation retorted, "There are more orthopaedic surgeons in Bangalore than at Baroda but we came here to get an expert hypnotherapeutic treatment". We cautioned we have never treated such a patient before. However, the patient did accept a different variety of skin grafts, not in common use by plastic surgeons now called pinch graft. When the first batch of pinch grafts succeeded after 4 sessions with hypnotherapy, we further covered the entire granulating surface with pinch grafts. The wound healed. Rheumatic gangrene is a highly complicated situation to a patient of rheumatoid arthritis. The rheumatic disease involves several organs including the heart, the vessels and other joints. When this can also be helped with hypnotherapy, our faith in ourselves was strengthened to treat other autoimmune disease also like Dermatomyositis, Multiple sclerosis, pemphigus, etc.

Amongst these, a case of pemphigus detected by a dentist while taking out a tooth is most significant. Pemphigus will affect the skin all over the body and may lead to death even. This was prevented by Dr. Sejal Thakkar.

Such instances are like a solitary cuckoo singing without a spring. But a scientific approach must reveal a mechanism of operation physiologically. It requires immense faith to surrender without any expectations of result. Such surrender to the Divine carries them forward through extensive disease like cancer or degenerative diseases.

With success with regards to autoimmune conditions, we focused on the unexplained reproductive failure. At the back of our mind, we were looking for psychodynamic factor that will contribute to impedance or even killing of the partner's sperm. This resulted in our publication of 3 papers by Dr. Rajni Vyas, a gynaecologist.

The Corona epidemic had an indirect contribution. So far the couples would need personal presence for hypnotherapy. When hypnotherapy was feasible with video conferences, we devised an app that the couple can use without the presence of therapist. Full details of this module are narrated in the next chapter.

Lata Hemchand, a practicing psychologist, invited us to NIMHANS. We held an advanced workshop for the professorial staff of NIMHANS where the head of the department of psychology, Prof. Dr. Kiran inaugurated. Dr. Ramchandra also presided all-throughout. Prof. Dr. Pasricha also attended most of the sessions. We knew that Dr. Pasricha had worked for several years with Ian Stevenson. She has a firm belief in incarnation after death. When we narrated a single incidence of taking a subject to her past life, craving for Krishna in this birth, she supported us firmly. When we tried to instil a kindle of hope that the patients will forget her craving for Krishna in about 6 months with affirmation, a neophyte of a Professor at NIMHANS retorted said, "We have invited you to teach us hypnotherapy. Don't teach us to tell lies!" When Prof. Pasricha told me later that, "When your intention was to kindle hope, that really works with a hypnotized subject to generate hope into a reality. Why did you have to apologize?" We pacified Prof.

Pasricha by quoting *Bhagavad Gita*, that a mature person should not enter into discussion with a neophyte.

We had quite a few visits from Canada by Dr. Kripa Thakur and Dr. Aruna Thakur. When Dr. Aruna appeared for her final MBBS examination, she broke all the records by securing all the prizes that are being offered. When the couple visited us, Dr. Aruna, now an eminent psychiatrist at Saskatoon, Canada, was happy that we are interested in hypnotherapy. But Dr. Aruna was a strict examiner. When she saw me treating a patient, she bluntly told me, "You will fail miserably." This cryptic remark was well compensated by Kripa Thakur.

Kripa Thakur was a master hypnotherapist. When he will treat a patient with menstrual disorder, the attending nurse will also start menstruating! But Kripa himself had an exam phobia. Dr. Aruna succeeded in getting the fellowship earlier and became the head of the department of psychiatry at Saskatoon.

Kripa Thakur explained to us as to how our hypnotherapy would be deficient without the appropriate use of metaphors and archetypal symbols. He said he belonged to Jabalpur in Madhya Pradesh where two eminent *Maharshis*[9] also found roots, namely Rajnish who later on became famous as Osho and Maharshi Maheshyogi, the founder of TM movement. So, Dr. Kripa explained that the appropriate use of archetypal symbols during hypnotherapy goes deep down into unconscious mind and the unconscious mind finds a way to work with these symbols just like Albert Einstein worked with symbols while deriving a mathematical proof for an equation!

Kripa Thakur fished out a book published in 1928 by a mathematician, Hadamard. He was researching the creative process in the mind of mathematicians. Mathematics involves progression with equations. Einstein in a typical fraternity bond that was usual for him replied to Hadamard which becomes a landmark for all creative processes. He wrote,

"My Dear Colleague:

In the following, I am trying to answer in brief your questions as well as I am able. I am not satisfied myself with those answers and I am willing to answer more questions if you believe this could be of any advantage for the very interesting and difficult work you have undertaken.

(a) The words or the language, as they are written or spoken, do not seem to play any role in my mechanism of thought. The psychical entities which seem to serve as elements in thought are certain signs and more or less clear images which can be "voluntarily" reproduced and combined. There is, of course, a certain connection between those elements and relevant logical concepts. It is also clear that the desire to arrive finally at logically connected concepts is the emotional basis of this rather vague play with the above-mentioned elements. But taken from a psychological viewpoint, this combinatory play seems to be the essential feature in productive thought—before there is any connection with logical construction in words or other kinds of signs which can be communicated to others.

(b) The above-mentioned elements are, in my case, of visual and some of muscular type. Conventional words or other signs have to be sought for laboriously only in a secondary stage, when the mentioned associative play is sufficiently established and can be reproduced at will.

(c) According to what has been said, the play with the mentioned elements is aimed to be analogous to certain logical connections one is searching for.

(d) Visual and motor. In a stage when words intervene at all, they are, in my case, purely auditive, but they interfere only in a secondary stage, as already mentioned.

(e) It seems to me that what you call full consciousness is a limit case which can never be fully accomplished. This seems to me connected with the fact called the narrowness of consciousness (Enge des Bewusstseins).

Remark: Professor Max Wertheimer has tried to investigate the distinction between mere associating or combining of reproducible elements and between understanding (organisches Begreifen); I cannot judge how far his psychological analysis catches the essential point."

We have taken recourse to the letter time and again. The reason to refer to this letter which to our mind is pristine, pure, precious than any jewel because here a twice awarded Nobel laureate connecting the creative process in a wholesome holistic manner. Even before neurolinguistic programming was first published Richard Bandler and John Grinder in 1975, Einstein has indirectly pointed that in his mathematical discoveries the usual language is not used and certain symbols, mainly visual, have played a role for programming. That points to a well established fact about creativity. Probably creativity is a descent from somewhere above, say Divinity, but the mysticism about creativity is thus well-documented.

Kripa Thakur explained how NLP should be used in programming a strategy for hypnotherapy. While every individual has five faculties in sensorium, he is more likely to be versatile in using any one particular sense. Having identified the most frequently used sensory faculty, say in case of Einstein, it was visual, and the strategy should revolve about structuring the design of a programme accordingly.

Our success in hypnotherapy is in that we design a specific programme for each individual just as a tailor-made suit fits better than a readymade one.

We have been time and again asked as to when you met Milton Erickson and how much time did you spend with him, etc. We have not followed Milton Erickson at all. The resemblance to our delivery may be in the eyes of the beholder.

Kripa Thakur explained to us as to how to induce metaphors in the strategy. Metaphors are the language of unconscious mind. They need not be explained because unconscious mind works in its own way to find a resolution that would have produced a symptom or a disorder or a disease. We like to illustrate with a real life situation:

A lady teacher teaching English in a English medium school was brought to us just for curiosity. When she asked that is there a solution for hypnotherapy with regards to migraine, we showed we are inclined to try. She volunteered there and then.

We asked her, "Please tell us what is the spelling of the word 'Fish'?"

"F-I-S-H"

"If I say, my dear proficient teacher in English, that you are wrong and the real spelling should be G-H-O-T-I?"

"Ghoti? I don't understand. That is the beauty of English language. Would you like to know why along with Bernard Shaw, we believe that the correct spelling should be Ghoti."

"How does Bernard Shaw figure in this dialogue?"

"That is the beauty when you will resolve your migraine with this dialogue."

"I do not understand... "

"Pun is most amazing when it is not explained but an English teacher does not understand this simple puzzle... "

"I am confused."

"For F in Fish, take Gh from rough, for I in Fish, take O from Women, and for sh in fish, take ti from nation."

The subject asked, "Why have y**ou to go** so far?"

"Because you have been carrying an unnecessary burden of an unresolved conflict that your unconscious mind has solved for you now. Your migraine is gone."

Gopa Guha is now carrying on as Hon. Editor of the newsletter of our Society without any migraine.

In conclusion, we assert that hypnotherapy is a science for sure. However, there are bad and excellent surgeons. So, there can be hypnotherapists which may fail to deliver.

Notes

1. Scriptures belonging to the late/post-Vedic period of Hinduism.
2. Oldest layer of Sanskrit scriptures in Hinduism.
3. Sages.
4. One of the four chapters in Patanjali's *Yoga Sutra.*
5. *Siddhis* are powers, abilities or attainments that are products of yogic advancements.
6. The ability to control the mind of others.
7. Poison damsel.
8. One that is beyond the boundaries of time.
9. Great sage.

2

Metaphors

What we are generally aware is our conscious mind that is as much visible as a tip of an iceberg. Mind consists of other 2 entities—subconscious mind that constitutes about 10%. Subconscious mind is what we can bring into attention with little deliberation. The iceberg that unconscious mind is, is the real driving force about which most of us are not aware. Yet, our everyday life is structured and manipulated by the drives from unconscious mind.

It will not be exaggeration to state that almost all of immature defences of the ego find expression through the different ego defences that are brought into force by the unconscious mind. When the fox gives up jumping after several attempts and tells itself that the grapes were sour, it has deployed immature defence of the ego so that he has protected himself from despair.

In addition to projection, Freud has described several immature defences of the ego. They are truly immature since the term indicates that in fact they are not real. They are: Acting out, Hypochondriasis, Passive-aggressive behaviour, Schizoid fantasy and splitting.

When a person develops a better perception to observe his own mind, he develops a reality perspective of the situation. Thereafter he has to continue to function in this world but he would do so with mature defences of ego.

Suppression of an unfulfilled desire by whatsoever mean so as not to yield to the irrational demands of id, was considered by Freud as mature defence of ego. In addition other mature defences of ego are anticipation, humour, sublimation and altruism.

Thus, according to Freud, an individual was constantly torn between the irrational demands of id and moral, ethical norms that dictate a decent social behaviour. Such a constant combat within oneself would not leave any room for peace. Most psychosomatic disorders arise from this trouble. This confirms the statement by father of *Ayurveda*, *Charaka* that almost all ailments arise out of the faulty functioning of the wisdom.

Modern medicine got illumined by the light of research by Hans Selye. Hans Selye as a medical student in Canada observed that rats subjected to severe cold as well as extreme heat exhibited a same group of syndromes that he termed as general adaptation syndromes. Now, modern medicine has advanced in understanding the stress response to the extent that the references to Selye by now exceed over 1000 patients as titles for the research work only. It brought to light that continuous stress for a prolonged period would lead to somatisation. That means that mental and emotional symptoms take the form of a particular disease. Long standing stress in the form of an unresolved conflict in the mind transforms into somatisation as per the attitude of the subject. A woman married maybe for 10+ years would not have noticed that she had congenital presence of cervical rib. This is an extra rib that has so far not caused any symptoms. Now that she has found it difficult to carry on the load on her shoulders due to stress, her radiology examination reveals for the first time that she has an extra rib. Frequently such a patient is subjected to major surgery for removal of the rib. That instantaneously takes off the symptoms of tingling and numbness that were generated due to the rib now pressing against the brachial plexus due to sagging muscles around the shoulders.

One such lady came to us to show the wonderful results obtained by removal of cervical rib. However, when we suggested to her that there may not be any need to undergo major surgery on another shoulder region provided she understands how stressfully she has been living with responsibilities of two young children, a bedridden mother-in-law with a joint family and carrying on a flourishing professional career. She differed the surgery. With recourse to physiotherapy, self hypnosis and adjusting the lifestyle so as to avoid excessive stress, she avoided surgery on another shoulder. Several instances may be recounted where excessive stress causes somatisation however; a classic situation is trigeminal neuralgia. Trigeminal nerve arises from a ganglion situated at the base of the skull in a perfectly well fitted location. When the Mesenchymal tissue in the ganglion that is swollen up due to large secretion of cortisol subsequent to persistent stress, there is sharp shooting pain on one side of the face that can be unbearable. Now an electronic device is available that can precisely localize the ganglion and destroy it. That leaves the patient without sensation. One of the students, a dentist, specialized in hypnotherapeutic stress removal so as to cure trigeminal neuralgia! Without going into the details of elaborate strategic hypnotherapy, we enumerate some of the other conditions that we have learnt to alleviate. They are: tennis elbow, ulcerative colitis, sciatica, frozen shoulder and culcaneal spur. We will further discuss the details as to how an illustrious saint in high order experienced somatisation of right shoulder. The shoulder was so frozen that he had continuous pain and limited movement. This is despite the fact that the saint was living in an ascetic frugal life. The therapy session was successful in relieving the pain that he was experiencing.

The saint as a blessing offered to Bhaskar Vyas an initiation into the order. We requested that this will be a blessing indeed if both of us, Rajni and Bhaskar, can be initiated jointly. The swami regretted since we had no authorization to initiate a lady.

It may be migraine as we have seen in the previous chapter, irritable bowel syndrome, phobias, etc. The link may extend to severe mental disorders like depression, schizoid tendencies and may progress to Parkinsonism. Persistent, long term stress can cause degeneration of a small segment of neurons. That is generally compensated by taking over the function by the adjacent neurons but such patchy numerous degenerations of neurons is said to be the root cause of Alzheimer's disease.

There are several ways whereby unconscious mind releases itself from the tensions generated because of stress. In addition to the defences enumerated earlier for the protection of ego, there are other windows like Freudian slip, dreams that generally express with metaphors or Freudian psychoanalysis. Freudian psychoanalysis was a favourite tool for psychologists as well as psychiatrists. It took several sessions extending into few months and yet there was no litmus test to prove that the stress is gone. On the other hand, hypnotherapy including advanced as hypnoanalysis has found an effective and the sessions can be concluded in 4-6 weeks. Sometimes, it also happens that the patient will experience a sudden bursting of insight in a single session or in a short time. Usually, a grateful patient may thank the therapist or a self asserting person that is the aim for all patients may eject the therapist, taking the entire credit for himself. That therapist would not mind, a hypnotherapist aims at the successful result with hypnotherapy; the credit for him is not the goal.

Further insight into the strategic planning of a session for hypnotherapy came in 1998 from Ernest Rossi. Prof. Ramchandra had planned a 7 day workshop along with 2 days conference. Ernest and his wife attended. He was an illustrious student of Milton Erickson. His therapeutic session lasted 90+ minutes, as per the dictates of Milton Erickson. This was one of the secrets of wonderful results by Erickson.

However, Ernest Rossi had an elegant hypothesis for genomic expressions during hypnosis process. No doubt, the entire protein synthesis is dependent on particular genes connected with that protein. The metaphor as utilized by Milton Erickson would definitely transform into the psychodynamic images as needed by the patient; but we have profound faith in Ernest Rossi and we believed that his hypothesis concerning the gene expression would also be provable. Rossi exhorted that we should take up some studies concerning genomics. Prof. Bharat Chattoo at M.S. University, Vadodara ruled it out as highly expensive. Collaborating with Prof. Dr. Nagaraja, at NIMHANS, we applied for a grant amounting to Rs. 6 crore from BIRAC.

Dr. Nagaraja was confident. We even planned to move to Bangalore. After presenting the proposal, BIRAC sent back to us a copy of the experts' reasons for rejection. One of them has considered it to be 'a huge wastage of public money'.

Yet, we were highly impressed by utilization of symbols based on the form of Devi Durga. Rossi hypothesized that within 2 minutes of hypnosis, 2 arms of Durga will start dancing. In another 20 minutes they will make entire 18 arms of Durga to dance. In the next 70 minutes or so, Devi Durga will dance in its full form so that an entire genome sequence relevant to the need of the patient may come into vogue.

Milton Erickson had no access to modern kind of laboratories. However, he was a brilliant philosopher who tried to understand fundamental basis of consciousness. In the process, he volunteered himself to take marijuana. The experiment is beautifully catalogued in the book, "Doors of Perception". This took Erickson to Aldous Huxley, a high profile philosopher of his times. In the last phase of their lives, they were collaborating together to arrive at synthesis of their research so that understanding of consciousness may progress. Unfortunately, Huxley's house where the manuscript was being stored got engulfed in a fire and the research is no more available.

What might be the form of archetypal symbols, deployed by Erickson is thus difficult to guess. Rossi's presentation with Devi Durga's moving 2 hands subsequently going to 18 and later on to a dance by the Devi was to have a poignant, permanent impression on our psyche. Durga traditionally holds the weapons of various gods of Hindu mythology, which they give her to fight the demon, *Mahishasur* since only a goddess will be able to slay him. She is depicted carrying a rosary, battle axe, mace, arrow, thunderbolt, lotus, bow, water pot, cudgel, lance, sword, shield, conch, bell, trident, goblet, noose and the sudarshan chakra[1] in 18 hands. The 18 armed form of Devi Durga is evoked only for destruction of evil.

These weapons are considered symbolic by Shakta Hindus, representing self-discipline, selfless service to others, self-examination, prayer, devotion, remembering her *mantras*, cheerfulness and meditation.

How do we contemplate to take hypnotherapy into archetypal symbols that may be rooted in the memory of the herd? We have found great relevance when story telling as derived from *Panchatantra, Ramayana, Mahabharata*, Birbal and Akbar's stories as well as the stories from '1001 Arabian Nights' have direct relevance to therapeutic success. This process we shall see in the next chapter.

Note

1 Divine discus.

3

Contemporizing Archetypal Symbols

Sometime back Bhaskar Vyas was diagnosed with Lymphoma. Lymphoma is a neoplastic growth that spreads slowly via lymphatic.

However, the prognosis for lymphoma is good with modern therapy. He was prescribed to have 10 sessions of deep X-ray to the pelvic region and spine. Thereafter, he had to take 6 intravenous injections of a recently developed drug as immune therapy once a month for 6 months.

To cover any adverse effects, including anaphylaxis, he was prescribed an intravenous injection of dexamethazone, half an hour before the injection of immune therapy. During the entire course of the treatment, he did not have a slightest side effect. This he attributes to excellent, strategic programme, specially designed for him. During the therapist's scholastic career, we had talked about Ernest Rossi and his presentation with the symbol of Devi Durga. The therapist used our axiomatic teaching to use the currency of the country. Though Bhaskar Vyas is not dedicated to any religious belief, the therapist knew his faith about Ernest Rossi. So, she deployed the symbol of Durga dressed in a brilliant red *sari*, with 4 hands. In one hand she had *trishul*/trident, in another she was holding a sickle, in the third she had a sword and in the fourth she had a conch. In one brilliant move, Devi Durga had been victorious in slaying the demon that was lymphoma and she was blowing the conch to celebrate the victory cry. The script of the session is as follows:

> "Make yourself as comfortable as possible. Whenever ... yes you may move any part of your body till you are in the most relaxed, comfortable and pleasing position. Whenever you choose to listen to this tape, find yourself some time where you will not be disturbed. Your own personal protected time. A place which is quiet, which is peaceful. A quiet, calm and peaceful place and once you are lying down or seated comfortably, Dr. Vyas, I request you to focus your attention. Focus your attention on my words and let us primarily change the surroundings. We may use the infinite potential of the mind to change the surroundings right here or if you wish or choose you may take your mind just drifting, a floating drifting or floating, flying to another place, another time. You find yourself now in a place which you are particularly fond of. A beautiful compound of a temple. Yes, you are outside the temple, you're sitting as you like it outside the temple. Perhaps on a bench, perhaps on a comfortable red bench in the courtyard and the time is early morning. In front of you is a temple. The temple may be of stone, carved out of stone with dedicated labour. Or perhaps it is a beautiful temple, a temple made of marble. Then again, only you can see it, perhaps it is made of bricks and cement and coloured and decorated in the most pleasing way but it is there, magnificent, majestic and beautiful. Yes, and you are out and God is within(2) and you are sitting outside and God is within, you are on the out and God is within. It's morning and the sun is warm, a soothing warmth, a comfortable warmth. Warmth which ferments your muscles. Makes you feel relaxed,

makes you feel comfortable. Yes, sitting so that the rays of the sun are fomenting your shoulders, your arms and various parts of your body. The sun is soft, warm and kind. There is also a breeze. A cool breeze cool and soft. Soft like the tender touch of a mother and the breeze. The breeze is caressing your head, your forehead like a gentle pat, hugging your shoulders, stroking your back like a warm, loving, fuzzy feeling that only a mother can give. The beautiful trees on the courtyard. Tall trees with multiple branches, full of wonderful green leaves. Leaves of tomorrow, leaves of hope, leaves of strength, leaves of growth, leaves of healing, leaves of repair, and from among the branches, the sun is falling to give light and shade. Light and shade. But neither is permanent. Places that are in shadow just now will soon be in light, yes. Places that are in the shade will soon be in the light. And you are sitting there, drinking in the calmness, the wonderful vibrations, the beauty around you, watching the birds pecking at some scattered seeds. They move their heads from side to side, peck around the seeds and perhaps they hop around and they flutter, they fly. What is the force in them, what is the energy? What is it that makes them move, or hop or flutter or fly? Sitting there on the bench, feeling the warmth and the coolness in front of the temple, outside the temple knowing that God is within, your eyes fall on the *dwaarpalakas*[1], the guardians and the gates of the temple. The *dwarpalakas* have a very important role as they stand guard to all the temples. Taking care of who and what they allow inside. Taking care to see even the select memories, the thoughts, the feelings, the emotions, allowing inside only... allowing inside only what is useful, what is healthy, what is productive. And yes, on this wonderful morning, as you sit in this courtyard knowing that God is within, knowing that

God is within you can hear the *mantra* being chanted. The reputation, the rhythm, a *mantra* that you like, a *mantra* that is full of meaning, it could be just an 'Aum' or it could be something else but it's being chanted, its being repeated and these is a soothing feeling that all this bring and as you make yourself comfortable on the bench, your ears are listening to the sounds, your skin is feeling comfortable, your mind is occupied in thoughts and yet the numerous processes going on all by themselves... *Apne aap*. (by it self)

The beating of your heart which is beating calmly, quietly and peacefully. Your breath, which is slow and deep, deep and slow. The digestion, the propulsion of food, numerous processes going on all by themselves and yet you know being a doctor, a therapist, a researcher, and a professor, you are fully aware that all you have to do, all you have to do is put a little attention, a little focus and you can make your skin warm up. You may make your skin warm up. You may make your muscle loose and relaxed. You may change the rhythm of the breathing making it most efficient, making it a slow deep parasympathetic state. You may change the heart and keep it a calm, quiet and peaceful heart. You just have to focus and you can bring about whatever you wish. Bring about a tremendous awakening and mobilization and energizing of various competent cells in your body. The macrophages, the monocytes, the neutrophils, the complement cascade, the NK cells, all you have to do is just put a little attention and as you are doing so, your breathing is going on and you may attend to your breathing if you wish, if you so choose you may focus on your breath at the level of the nose feeling and sensing, sensing and feeling and experiencing the movement of air in and out of your nose perhaps noticing that the air that you exhale, the air that you breath out is a little warmer than the air that you breathe in. Perhaps noticing the *Dwarapalakas* right there in the nose in the form of tiny tiny hair, or special chemicals in the mucus that keep out all that's unwanted. Unwanted regrets, unwanted sadness, unwanted anger. You may focus at the level of the nose or if you wish, if you choose, you may quietly observe the gentle rise and fall of your chest. Or using the infinite potential of the mind, you may follow the breath from the nose, to the pharynx to the windpipe all the way down to the alveoli, where the inate wisdom, the intelligence that your body already possesses, chooses, takes in the life giving oxygen. This oxygen travels all the way down to the tips of your toes, all the way to the top of your head and all the way across to the tip of your fingers. Soothing, relaxing and yet energizing and mobilizing all the immunocompetent cells. Breathing in oxygen, breathing in the positivity, breathing in all the blessings of the masters and breathing out carbon dioxide, breathing out unwanted thoughts, unwanted feelings, and unwanted behaviours. Yes, you may focus on your breath, breathing in and out, in and out, and I wonder if you have heard of breathing into the heart, breathing gratitude into the heart. Breathing in a feeling of gratitude deep into your heart and breathing out and allowing the gratitude to mingle and merge with every cell in your body for there is no better emotion, no better state than a state of complete gratitude, when the homeostasis is perfect, when the hormones, the neurochemicals, the neuropeptides and all the physiology and the biochemistry is at its perfect working state and gratitude for the numerous blessings, for the wonderful moments. Your birth as a healthy boy... a boy, a gender of choice in a country where it matters, completely healthy in a loving family. Food and security and shelter and clothes, and opportunities to study, to live, to evolve, to learn, to grow, and acquirement of skills after skills as you became a doctor, a surgeon, a professor, a researcher and even a social worker. Being the medium of empowering so many people, of travelling to many places, of being treated with respect, of being felicitated, the wonderful moments, the blessings, the achievements, the moments of smile, the moments of curious learning, the moments of satisfaction, allow this feeling of completeness, the feelings of adequacy, the feelings of fullness to fill your heart and reach every place in your body. Breathing in and breathing out gratitude. As you sit there in the courtyard on the red bench listening to my voice, you have numerous choices, every second, every millisecond, every fraction of a moment, we are making choices. Sometimes consciously, sometimes unknowingly. You may choose to simply hear my voice... just keeping on hearing my voice. But then again you may choose to focus on my words or you may choose to wonder, to ponder about the meanings of my lines and then again if you were to choose, if you were to choose, if you were to choose to not focus on my words, not focus on the words but on the pause. On the gap. On the space between my words, you will find the space, this pause, this gap to be full of peace, quiet and this soothing silence. Peace and quiet and a soothing silence that is spreading all around you... all around you and slowly, slowly, slowly into you. Peace, quiet and a soothing silence. Yes... you can focus on your breath, you can breathe in gratitude all the while holding on to my voice and as you sit or lie down, now your eyes are closed, your eyelids are relaxed, your eyelids are sitting quietly as if they are stuck to your eyes. When our eyes are open, when our eyes are wide, wide open, what do we see? You know and I know and we all know that when our eyes are wide, wide open, we can see all around us. We can see what's in front of us, what's beside us, what's above us, what's below us, we may even turn and see what's behind us and what do we see when our eyes are closed and our lids are sitting relaxed on top of our eyes, what do we see then? We choose and select and we can see any image, any picture, any visual, or any movie of our own personal choice. Like right now. Perhaps you are beholding, perhaps you are visualizing, and perhaps you can see the glorious image, the beautiful image of Goddess Durga. Goddess Durga in all her glory, sitting on the tiger, with the hair, her dark black cascading hair, the *mukut*[2] on her head, the golden crown on her head, a beautiful red *sari* with a golden border. There she is. A beautiful image with various ornaments, with garlands, vision of immense beauty, a sparkling glorious divine image and as you look at her do you see 2 hands or 4 hands or 8 hands or 16 hands! And what do they hold? Do they hold the *trishul*, do they hold a *dhanushya* and a *teer*, do they hold a sickle, do they hold a conch, do they hold the *sudarshan chakra*? What are these numerous weapons? What are they the tools of? They are the tools to destroy, to get rid of unwanted demons. Unwanted demons, for isn't she *Mahishasurmardini*[3]? The killer of Mahishasur and Mahishasur may be anything, it may be an unwanted memory an unwanted thought, an unwanted emotion or an unwanted patch of cells. But there she is. A warrior, a wise, wise warrior. A warrior with valour and wisdom who is always victorious. A wise victorious brave warrior. And she exists or the demon exists and where she exists and she exists in every X chromosome, in every cell of your body, there she is—*Shakti*. The most strong, powerful strength, the *Brahman*. There she is, in every cell in your body, energizing, mobilizing, and bringing about a movement. Feel and sense her presence. Feel and sense the inner strength. Feel and sense the strength, the confidence, the valour, the boldness as the divine light courses through your veins, through your lymphatic, through various vessels in your body. Taking care of you, protecting you, keeping you safe. She is the warrior queen, but she is also a mother; your mother, my mother, everyone's mother. Birth after birth, every single birth a mother looking after us with kindness, with love, with compassion and affection. Feel her presence in the very core of your being and with every breath that you breathe in, you are breathing in calm, breathing in quiet, breathing in peace and every time you breathe out, you are breathing out your doubts, you are breathing out your fears. Yes, and you can stretch out and make yourself even more comfortable. Perhaps cover yourself with a soothing, relaxing blanket, a magical blanket, a relaxing blanket, a healing soothing relaxing blanket. You can choose the texture, you can choose the material. It may be simple cotton, or a warm woolly blanket or smooth silky silk. You can have it in your favourite colour. It may be plain or it may have some design on it. But this blanket is no ordinary blanket and as you cover your body from the toes to the shoulders, all the way up this blanket. Wherever the blanket touches your body, that part of your body becomes completely relaxed. You may visualize, you may sense, you may feel the blanket touching the 10 little toes of your feet and with the tender touch, the toes are becoming loose and relaxed. All the toes on your feet, you can see it, you can sense it, and you can feel it. And this soothing blanket, this healing blanket, this remarkable blanket with magical properties is moving over your feet. Sliding and gliding over the tired muscles of your feet and under the touch of the blanket, this magical blanket, this healing blanket, your feet muscles are becoming loose and relaxed so that now your toes are relaxed, your feet are relaxed and your mind is supremely calm (2) and then the blanket is moving up, having relaxed your toes, relaxed your feet, its moving over your ankle joints and moving up inch by inch, *dheere dheere se*[4], little by little, up your leg towards your knees. Relaxing the leg muscles, relaxing the calf muscles so that you feel a comfortable feeling in your legs. Relaxing your leg muscles, giving comfort and a pleasing sensation to your legs. Yes, your toes they are relaxed, your feet are relaxed, your ankles relaxed, your calf muscles very comfortable and your mind is supremely calm, quiet, peaceful and patient. The blanket is moving over your knee joint relaxing both your knees and as it relaxes your knees, it also sends healing vibrations over your mind. Restoring health, repairing healing, restoring normalcy to both your knees so that your toes they are relaxed, your feet are relaxed, your ankles are relaxed, your leg muscles are relaxing now, your knees are relaxing. Your mind is supremely *shaant*[5], *sthir*[6], calm, quiet and peaceful. The blanket is now moving further up over your thighs, relaxing your thighs and the bigger muscles, the thigh muscles are becoming very comfortably relaxed and you are feeling a nice comfortable sensation. And then blanket moves over your hip region, over your pelvic region. This is no ordinary blanket, it's a magical blanket and it sends waves inside, restoring normalcy, getting rid of any unwanted cells, any unwanted muscles, restoring total, and complete health. Then it moves over your abdominal region, relaxing your abdominal muscles, making sure that the right level of enzymes, of acid, right level of insulin, right level of sugar in your blood, then it moves up over your chest. Relaxing the muscles of your chest, relaxing the muscles of your chest and your breathing is becoming deep and slow or perhaps it is becoming slow and deep. Breathing in oxygen, breathing in confidence, breathing in courage, breathing in inner strength, breathing out carbon dioxide, breathing out your worries, your doubts, your fears and your heart is beating quietly now. Your heart is beating peacefully. Your heart is beating calmly, quietly, peacefully, with regular rhythm. The blanket has come to your shoulders and the shoulder muscles are relaxing and it's a wonderful feeling, a soothing feeling of comfort. A very pleasing feeling. It's like you are adding more and more water to clay and the clay becomes really loose and the shoulder muscles are becoming very loose and comfortable and this soothing comfort, this soothing comfort is flowing into your arms from the shoulders up to the elbows, relaxing your arm muscles, relaxing your elbows, relaxing your forearm muscles, relaxing your wrist, relaxing all the muscles till the tip of your fingers till both your hands are completely relaxed and the blanket stops here at the level of the shoulders. Tiny, tiny waves of relaxation are spreading up along the ribbon like muscles of your neck. To relax your chin, relax your facial muscles, relax the small muscles around your mouth, relax the tiny muscles around your nose. Relax your forehead. Relaxing all your facial muscles till your face resembles that of a young baby without a single crease without a single furrow, smooth, carefree, *nishchint*[7], *befikar*[8], lying safely, sleeping peacefully in the lap of mother. And this is how you are feeling now, relaxed, carefree, safe, light. And in this feeling of safety and comfort, all the internal processes are in perfect harmony. The tiny waves, the waves of relaxation are spreading to your scalp, relaxing your scalp muscles, bringing soothing comfort to your head and cascading like a waterfall down your back, relaxing all the muscles along the back. Back of head, back of neck, back of shoulders, upper back, middle back, lower back, back of hips, back of thighs, back of knees, back of legs, all the way down till every muscle is relaxed. Every muscle is relaxed, every joint is relaxed. The sympathetic are quiet; it's a state of rest and relax. There are no enemy neurochemicals now. The immune system is wide awake, it's alert, it's fully awake, it's in peak energy, it's in total energy, highly energized to fight off any irregular happening. And as your mind is much calmer state than what it was and as your body is more relaxed, whatever I speak to you, whatever I tell you, whatever I speak will go into the deep, deep layers of your unconscious mind, much like salt dissolves in water and your thoughts, your emotions and your actions will be greatly influenced by what I say. As we go through the motions of living, with the purpose of being effective. What could be effective mean? Doing what is required, doing what is necessary, irrespective of whatever our emotions may be, standing with a bat and hitting every ball that comes our way, mindfully, living in the moment with complete awareness. Managing the moments, the milliseconds, the minutes, the hours, the days, the weeks. Yes, and slowly as we travel through life's way, just like when it's time for a flower to become a fruit, the petals give way. The petals drop one by one. The petals of attachment, the petals of excessive desire, the petals of ego identification and then we know that the petals are dropping and this flower is going to become a fruit. Breathing in calm, breathing out and relaxing. Breathing in peace, breathing out and relaxing. Breathing in quiet, breathing out and relaxing and in this relaxed state, perhaps I can tell you a story of a sage. A sage called Markandeya and he lived in the Himalayas, along the banks of a beautiful river in a valley and this river was called Pushpabhadhra. And this sage was in a state of equipoise. He lived a very severe austere life with tremendous discipline. His mind, his body, his intellect, totally in his control, identifying with the *Aatman* and as he did so, he became extremely powerful and Lord Indra felt very insecure and said "What if this sage tries to take my place? What if this sage tries to become the next Indra?" And because of his insecurities, he sent numerous beautiful ladies—nymphs, slim, wearing beautiful flowing garments, with flowers in their hair. He also hired Kamadev to strike the sage with his bow and arrow and the music rose and the nymphs danced and the clothes fell off and the hair hung loose and the fragrant flowers were everywhere, but all this, including Kamadev was waiting with his bow and arrow, hardly disturbed the sage. And when it reached the crescendo, the sage opened his eyes, and so much was his power, so much was his Divine energy, so much was his power of realizing his true state of identifying with the *Aatman*[9] that Kamadev and the nymphs and the celestial being had to run far away to save their lives. This is the story. When God comes and asks him, what boon do you wish? And Markandeya says, I have never experienced *Maya*, do tell me what this is? What is this thing that you people call *Maya*[10]? And this is just a story and you are sitting on the bench in the courtyard listening to my voice and breathing in, breathing out and relaxing and while your body continues to breathe out, expelling carbon dioxide, expelling unwanted doubts, unwanted fears, and unwanted worries. Relaxing further and further, relaxing more and more, you can take the infinite power of your mind to make another journey to another place at another time. And now you find yourself, the time is a beautiful evening and you are walking at the seashore another place that you love. The vast, vast apparently limitless sea. You are walking and your feet can feel the sand. Its granular, it's coarse, at places it's dry and at some places it's moist and at some places it's even wet. You are walking barefoot and every step leaves a footprint. Every step changes the shape of the sand. You can see tall, tall coconut trees and what drives the sap all the way up to the leaves. You are looking at the coconut trees, your ears are listening to the rhythmic sound of the waves. The waves as they come and recede, come and go. Your eyes can appreciate the beautiful sky, the evening sky. The evening sky with a mixture of colours, of yellow, your favourite orange, red, gold, white and blue. It's like a beautiful canvas of wonderful mixture of colours. Your eyes are drinking in the colours, your ears are listening to the sound of the waves. Your skin is feeling the touch of breeze. Your feet are in touch with the sand and you can go perhaps to the edge of the water and watch the white foamy waves, feel the sprinkling of water on your face, and allow all your unwanted emotions, the emotions heighten the adrenaline, that heighten the cortisol, let these unwanted memories, the unfinished business, the unwanted thoughts, allow them to descend from your brain box to your chest to your abdomen to your thighs to your heel to your toes to be washed away (2), to the bottom of the sea. Leaving you light, leaving you free, and leaving you like a new slate. And you are feeling much more energetic now, much more comfortable now, more happy now, more joyous now, and with this newly freed energy, this newly freed energy you are making more brisker steps on the beach, walking with more brisk steps till you come to a beautiful sand castle. It's an amazing sand castle, so beautifully made, with skill, with patience, you are appreciating the beauty of the castle when a massive wave comes and washes it away. It was just *Maya*, it was just delusion, and it's gone. The sand is there, the form is different. The sand lies now partially in the water, partially on the beach. You are walking further on, looking at the sky, observing the sun, the sun is in the west, it's round, it's orange, and just before drops at the horizon, hides behind the sea, it takes in all your unfinished emotions, whatever emotions are there, whatever tiny remnants of anger or sadness or regrets, it takes all that in, becomes a fiery red and hides at the horizon and yes it will come up again with a new name. It will call itself a new day. As the sun dips behind the sea, as the sun hides behind the sea, it has left you even more free than before, more light, more energetic, more joyous, and your blood pressure, your sugar levels, your hormones, your immunocompetent cells, everything are just as they should be—in homeostasis. A perfect biochemistry, a perfect physiology. The moon is slowly coming up. Others at the beach are moving to their homes. There is an atmosphere of peace, an atmosphere of calm. So calm, so peaceful, the moon is spreading its milky white moonlight so that the moonlight is making the waves shimmer. Making the sand look a beautiful white colour. It is also cleansing you, bathing you, wiping you, renewing you, a cool, cool light as patience, as tolerance, as forgiveness and compassion arise in you, arise and flow through your body. Love, patience, compassion, forgiveness, feeling every cell moving through your vessels, moving through your lymphatic. You're looking up at the moon now. The moon, does it have its own light or does it borrow the light? Whom does it borrow the light from and in this moment of questioning and wonder and curiosity and you are looking at the sea but the waves are fading away and giving way to a sea of light. You are looking at the trees but the margins are disappearing, and there's just light, you are looking at the sky but you cannot see the sky anymore. You cannot see your body anymore, there's just light. A tremendous light that fill everywhere, that's outside, that's inside, that is up that is below, there is nothing but light. What is this? Without a beginning, without an end, which is so subtle yet all pervading. What could this be? Yes, an awakening. An awakening and a blossoming. A blossoming at the top of your head of a thousand petal lotus. A violet lotus and you, where in this position there is no thought, there is no speech, there is thus the identification. Your true being of who you are, you are the *aatman*, you are the divine, you are the God and nothing. All the things that come and go are just a delusion. And you go on without a beginning without an end, you are everywhere. The 'I' that always goes on and then they all come back. You can see the sea now. You can see the sky now. You can see the clouds. The sky is vast and blue. The sea is a beautiful sea green, the clouds are pure white and move softly. Drift slowly but you have changed. The caterpillar has become a butterfly. The seed has turned into a sapling. Changes have occurred and these changes, so that everything is the same yet you know that nothing can be the same again. This divine experience has brought about an immense change in your mind, in your intellect, in your body and your heart. Your mind returns to where you were sitting. There on a bench. A red bench (3) in the courtyard where you are sitting outside. You are outside knowing the God is within. That the divine forces are within. And if I ask you where are you? Will you say that I am sitting on a bench and this bench is in a courtyard. This courtyard of a temple. The temple in this location, in this state, in this country, on this continent, on Earth, in this galaxy and all the galaxies in the lap of Goddess Durga as she smiles looking over you, taking care of you with loving motherly emotions. Protecting you, wherever you may be whichever moment, every step of the way. Taking all these images, these feelings of peace, these feelings of comfort. With

> the divine energy coursing through your vessels, your veins, your lymphatic, the mind is slowly coming back to where your body is resting and relaxing here on the bed. I shall slowly count from the count of 10 to the count of 1 and after the count of 1, whenever you feel ready, you may open your eyes. 10... Feeling calm and relaxed even when you are not listening to my voice 9.8.7.6... The flower that's giving way, dropping the petal one by one and finding its true identity and 5.4.3.2... feeling relaxed, feeling calm, feeling patient, having the perfect state of healing and repair 1. Whenever you feel ready, and it's been an amazing privilege and I thank you for allowing me to conduct this session. Thank you for the faith, thank you for the honour."

Of course the modern medical therapy is effective against lymphoma. However, oncotherapists advised one more PET scan to rule out the presence of any neoplastic cells that could have escaped. This was declined by the patient. Thereafter, we have time and again taken recourse to deployment of symbolic deities as per the belief of the patient.

Recently an alcohol addict, retired from air force, asked therapy to give up alcohol. When asked what his motive is when he has been drinking for 30 long years, he answered that Gujarat is a dry state. There is a social stigma associated with drinking and moreover with advancing age, he wants to protect his liver. On detailed interrogation, he revealed that for protection he has profound faith in Lord Hanuman.

The first session was designed with recitation as prayer for Hanuman. The subject instantaneously happened to go into deep trance without any formal induction. Thereafter, the subject gave up alcohol for good. But as therapists and for the witnessing students, this generated a double validity. Our axiomatic teaching that we should use appropriate symbols as per the belief system of the patient—currency of the country as an idiom—had been demonstrated successfully. Second thing, *Hanuman Chalisa*[11] had to be sung as a devotional song which was a successful demonstration of utilization of music as an induction strategy as well as therapy. Following detailing as an explanation that we have occasionally used music as a sole strategic therapy, a dermatologist doctor working at AIIMS, Delhi, wanted facilitation when she will want to do a PhD with music as a sole induction and therapeutic strategy.

PhD as a degree from any University would be the highest academic qualification. Yet, the novice therapists Richard Bandler and John Grinder have with their seminal publication earned the distinction for putting NLP as one of the strategies.

Similar to Bandler and Grinder, Ulf Sandstrom and his team has contemporized NLP further with only use of a touch and no language. They first used it when they set out on a ship to help the widows of civil war in Rwanda. On arrival there, they found difficulty with language. Hence, these innovations as Trauma Tapping Technique with the use of only touch.

Through their work with traumatized populations in the Peaceful Heart Network since 2007 they offered simple and efficient techniques for regulating symptoms of stress and trauma. The number one technique was the Trauma Tapping Technique - TTT derived from Thought Field Therapy and developed specifically for working with trauma peer to peer.

With TTT you activate the parasympathetic nervous system by tapping acupressure points on the hands, chest and on the face. To do the tapping takes about 5 minutes.

Results can vary from immediate changes to overnight shifts, and for some a small relief. For some the stress in prison and refugee camps is so high that it becomes a temporary relief, and for them it is useful to learn how to self-regulate. For this, instructions for "homework" are given in printed form and/or as the free app: Self Help for Trauma.

Symptoms of stress that commonly are relieved include anxiety, heart palpitation, sleep issues, headaches (stress related), stomach issues, hypervigilance, panic and racing thoughts.

For those with traumatic memories that are activated during treatment TTT can provide both temporary relief, and at times also resolve reactions completely in 1-3 sessions. This is what is called memory reconsolidation and amygdala depotentiation.

TTT can be taught in groups, learned as a self help, and in some cases needs to be facilitated by somebody.

TTT has been taught in over 30 countries, including to survivors of the genocide in Rwanda, liberated child soldier in Democratic Republic of Congo and survivors of the earthquakes and torrential rains in Nepal. The following figure shows the points for TTT technique:

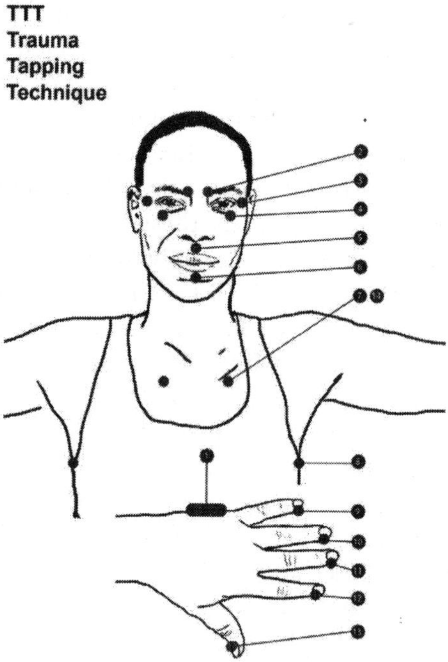

1. Medial side of the palm
2. Eyebrows
3. Lateral angle of the eye
4. Under the eye
5. Above the lips in the midline
6. Below the lips
7. And 14. Below the clavicle on the left and right side
8. Under the armpits
9. 9 to 13 Fingertips of the hands.

Dr. Pankhuri has yet to finish her fellowship at Oxford. So, the innovator should follow her own instinct.

We have successfully used music as induction technique and as a therapeutic strategy. We have not published so far. So whatever route Dr. Pankhuri may choose, we will like her name to go in the annals of hypnotherapy as one who contemporized music therapy in modern times.

The innovators have provided enough proofs on the basis of neuroscience. However, we take music as a therapy even up to the ancient times. We first utilized *Raga*[12] *Malkauns* known as *Hindolam* in South India. A patient from Saudi Arabia arrived with a diagnosis stamped by a psychiatrist as depression. When she walked in our room, we instantly diagnosed that her total demeanour is not indicative of depressive illness. On detailed interrogation, it was surprising to know that she has not witnessed any moment of joy.

> When asked about marriage,
> "My parents got me married since daughters have to be married when they are adults."
> "What about sex?"
> "A married woman is supposed to yield to the demand of her husband."
> "What about having two babies?"
> "The childbirth is a painful process. That's a biological disadvantage every woman is supposed to reconcile with."

This kind of counselling advice was of no avail. She was a highly intelligent, left-brain oriented person, impossible to even to put to hypnosis even with our favourite confusion technique. However, when we took her to her school days, she opened up to say that she enjoyed group singing. Yet, the subject of the music was not prayer. Her parents were both the members of communist party. Communists do not believe in God. When taken further she has to yield that the aesthetics is the soul of music and she had sung *Raga Malkauns* in her school days.

This was the first time we deployed music as an induction technique. Together we sang *Raga Malkauns* and she went into deep hypnosis with age regression. On waking up, she confessed for the first time that she had enjoyed what is true joy! With four more sessions of music therapy, she went back to Saudi Arabia fully satisfied. As an evident proof she brought her husband and two children to present sweets to us.

Raga Malkauns is an ancient *Raga* credited to be first innovated by Parvati, consort of Lord Shiva. Lord Shiva was fuming with anger when his meditation was interrupted by an arrow from Kaamdev. Kaamdev was instructed by Lord of all Devas, Indra, since he misunderstood that with profound meditation, Lord Shiva will become more powerful than him. Regardless, Shiva was about to burn out Kaamdev with opening of his third eye. If this were to happen, there will be no life on the Earth. That time, Devi Parvati came to help by first singing *Raga Malkauns* that put Shankara's wrath to cool down. Thus *Malkauns* has an essential property of being highly pleasing, destroyer of anger and creator of joy.

Deepak Raja, a sitarist himself, is better known by his deciphering the properties of various *Ragas.* The properties he has translated as *Raga-ness*, but further discussion with several *Ragas,* he puts into grammar so as to produce a specific feature. "The Raga-Ness of Ragas: Ragas Beyond the Grammar"—Deepak Raja.

Dr. Avnish Dave, now the Dean of a medical college, has yet another dimension to add to contemporization from ancient tradition. Ancient tradition has stipulated that at the root of the spine, there is a serpent like plexus called *kundalini.* This was supposed to be a seat of dormant energy that can be released by the practitioners of *Hath Yoga.* Ascending upwards, there are 7 nerve plexuses or *chakras* beginning from *Muladhara Chakra*—Root Chakra, *Svadhishthana Chakra*—Sacral Chakra, *Manipura Chakra*—Solar Plexus Chakra, *Anahata Chakra*—Heart Chakra, *Vishuddha Chakra*—Throat Chakra, *Ajna Chakra*—Third Eye Chakra, *Sahasrar Chakra*—Crown Chakra. It is well established that such nerve plexuses do exist in the body. Moreover, autonomic nervous system is regulated autonomously only by silent commands from vagus nerve and sympathetic ganglia. So there is a well established anatomical fact as well as physiological control by autonomic nervous system. That intense nerve plexuses that constitute the *chakras*, are well hypothesized by *Tantric* tradition. A hypnotherapist believes that he has access to unconscious mind through these *chakras*.

When modern oncotherapy for lymphoma was over in the first phase, we asked Dr. Avnish Dave to invoke all 7 *chakras* into action whereby our belief that the lymphoma has been vanquished is strengthened. Dr. Dave crafted an elegant session that will contemporize ancient tradition to present age.

We now revert back to a philosophical perspective. That was taught by Rohit Mehta. During the last year of his life, he emphasized that creative visualization is the substantiative basis for materialization of any idea. Of course even Plato has said that idea is the first reality but Kashmir Shiva Agamas have provided a blueprint. Unfortunately, the *pundits* of this Shiva Agamas are now a rarity. Yet, we studied two books by Jaideva Singh, 'Siva Sutras: Yoga of supreme identity' and 'Vijnanabhairava: Divine consciousnesses'. The books providing high erudition may not suit the modern young reader in search of instant remedies. Yet, the essence prevails. *Siva Sutras* postulate that there are 2 fundamental driving forces in the universe. 1. Creative power of thought: *Icchashakti* and 2. Formative power of thought: *Kriyashakti* Creative power primarily resides within several synaptic connections that intermingle and create a matrix that maybe a unique innovation or a reproduction of something that has already happened. When this matrix gels into a fabric, there is birth of an idea. In a hypnotic state, the idea may be seen as a symbol, as Einstein did, or it may take any of the forms as per neurolinguistic sensibilities of the therapist.

In 1987, Rohit Mehta inaugurated Baroda Hypnosis Society at Vadodara. He was not a hypnotherapist, Rohit Mehta was a philosopher, not only in the Western sense but what a philosopher would be called in Sanskrit and most Indian languages, he was a

Darshanik.[13] Such a philosopher sees the obvious truth as if it was descending way down before his eyes as a Divine Bliss. The *Gita* calls this kind of intuition as *Daivam.*[14] So, the ideas descend through the intervention of Divine deity, *Icchashakti* that is creative power of thought. However, it is enjoined up on each hypnotherapist that to a patient he would give the direction through invocation of the divine powers that may be residing in the brain of the patient. The therapist thereafter has a further duty to provide a roadmap to recovery. However, the therapist must deploy much wisdom as to what are the inherent capabilities of each individual. According to Abraham Maslow, an individual is capable of self-actualization that means whatever are the innate, inherent possibilities in the formation of that unique human being.

At that occasion, he explored the limitless possibilities that hypnotherapeutic strategies unfold. He said about how the formative power of thought comes into operation thus: Experimental and clinical psychologists have proved beyond a shadow of doubt that human nervous system cannot tell the difference between an actual experience and an experience imagined vividly and in detail. If the human nervous system cannot make a difference between the two, then the brain would immediately start functioning with regard to the impacts that come from something imagined in the same way it would do if something were actually happening.

When the idea thereafter is instilled in the trance state of a patient, he is given full freedom, maybe of 359 degrees to generate a format as per his sensibilities. The subject is encouraged to dream far and wide and vast and immense. However, the materialization into actuality will be limited only by the circumstances of the situation. Small or big, the formative power of thought has the potential to actualization. Once an idea takes deep roots into the unconscious mind, it formulates its own strategy as to how material achievement has to be achieved. We have deployed this strategy so as to fundamentally carve the idea into unconscious mind. As a final step in therapy, we employ future projections as being visualized by the hypnotized subject; witnessing the divine dance of two creative deities has provided succour to many of our patients diagnosed with depression. Thus, the panoramic vista of hypnotherapy is immensely vast and its aesthetic beauty shall depend on the view of the craftsman.

Success of hypnotherapy depends very much on the sensibilities of the patient as well as expertise of the therapist; the soil and the seed are both important yet a therapist endowed with a vast repertoire of stories as archetypal symbols can cultivate the ambience so as to achieve better results year after year and decade after decade. Milton Erickson has done so much for hypnotherapy. His success is still available to the novice so as to use river, sea, mountains, hills, trees, forests, and the leaves, etc. as archetypal symbols. What Freud elucidated in his masterpiece as 'Interpretation of Dreams' in 1899 is still relevant to entire mankind and maybe utilized as symbols in trance. Yet, the 21st century demands a further contemporization that is the relevance of this book.

Case 1 History: Brahmeshananda Swami—Age-65years

Complained of right frozen shoulder. He was a medical doctor specialized in gastroenterology and was giving honorary service in Ramakrishna Mission Hospital in Varanasi. He would be busy dispersing his knowledge and would treat more than 100 cases a day. Being Swamiji for more than 40 years, he would have his daily meditation practice plus medical practice. He was well adjusted and happy to be doing this routine day in and out.

He was given a new assignment. From being very active in his practice of medicine, he was posted on a table job to act as an editor of 70 years old journal on spirituality. Very soon he developed this complaint of being unable to use his right hand. Being a medical doctor, he tried to assess his frozen shoulder with allopathic investigations and explanation. Being a meditator, he approached us and we treated him with hypnotherapy and he was functional.

Brief

Swamiji, Hypnosis acts at a psychic level, at the unconscious mind which is the most powerful driving force. Neither Swamiji nor me nor anybody around has any need to know where the shoe pinches. It's totally different from psychoanalysis. It has nothing to do with analysis, whatsoever, it primarily generates insight. One gets insight through meditation, one gets insight through hypnosis. There is a Ramkrishna Paramhansa in all of us.

So Swamiji, I will begin my session with *Pranprathisthan.*[15] I will pray for 2 minutes all by myself and I will expect Swamiji to go into a state of *Turya*[16] in whatever maybe your way. Kindly allow me to touch you on your hands, arms and shoulders. Then I will ask for your permission, I have got a hypodermic needle with me which is to test whether the treatment is efficacious. So if Swamiji permits me to use the hypodermic needle then I am using it.

Session

Swamiji is deeply relaxed and with this *Pranprathisthan* I invoke, I invoke all the healing, Swamiji let go, deep deep breathing (2), and with each deep breath Swamiji is in, has entered a state of profound meditation, so easy Swamiji as I touch your right hand, see how profoundly you have relaxed yourself, your right hand falls like a stone. Your left hand falls like a stone and in this state of profound, intense, let go. Swamiji in wriggling his toes, wriggle your toes Swamiji.

Now so profound you are relaxed Swamiji, for someone who has been in the constant presence of Ramkrishna Paramhansa, Maa Sardadevi, Swami Vivekananda and the divinity itself, let go, who has served the afflicted relentlessly for all the years, who is so relieving the *kleshas*[17] of numerous innumerable one and the only Narayana as I touch your forehead Swamiji, one who has seen the one and only one Narayana and you have been face to face, face to face with *Daridra Narayana*[18] and that Narayana who dwells in the stomach of the hungry and the deprived one,

Swamiji, it has been your privilege and so you have been blessed by the Narayana himself. Yes Swamiji your right hand is your Yes hand and shall we say your left hand is your No hand. And as you take a further and deeper and deeper breath you have entered a state of profound trance and having entered a state of profound trance all other sounds except my voice and the eternal sound OM humming through your heart, the various centres of your brain and each and every cell of Swamiji's body, the eternal healing primordial sound of OM, OM. OM... is being heard, everything else is fading far far away. When Swamiji is now hearing the primordial healing sound of OM. Yes, Swamiji yes hand has moved and told me and in your listening, in your humming we too Swamiji and myself and others we who are here, we all are blessed to hear the eternal healing sound OM. That is now reverberating all around. And in this very reverberation of the energy perfectly alright to throw away all the irritations, all the *kleshas* and okay to cough them out if there be a need, in the universal healing process of OM reverberation. The *kleshas* have to just fade away and as they fade away Swamiji is further letting go of the aided and the emancipated who has healed, cured and salvaged so many, that in that very salvation, you are going through a rapid process of seeing all those faces, Swamiji, the deprived, the depraved, the sick and the suffering whom you helped and as you see their faces in a rapid succession of like a fast forward video filming you see the immutable face of Narayana and as you think this face of Narayana your right thumb moves. The face of Narayana is face to face with Swami Brahmeshananada and that is the natural due of Swamiji.

Swamiji any of the finger or the thumb of your right hand moves. Yes Swamiji when you move this, the face becomes clearer and clearer, further clearer. Your right hand is so comfortable, profound state of peace, tranquillity and serenity is all over all over the mind, body and let go relaxed wonderful. What a divine flash of light. How profoundly illuminated as you swallow that saliva Swamiji. It has given me as much peace and happiness as to see Ramkrishna Paramhansa himself and eating and drinking by himself. Perfectly our due to scratch away all the afflictions that may be on the surface of the nose or within the deeper recesses, the mind in such a way that the *kleshas* are transforming themselves into *akleshas*[19] in relieving the suffering of the arduous, Swamiji has accumulated so much of that affliction, wriggling himself that Swamiji needs to do a bit of further work now, Swamiji so that we get rid of those accumulated afflictions acquired by others, i.e. Swamiji's natural due.

Would Swamiji, yes when you want to do that extra bit of work, thank you for saying yes. It's my privilege to serve you who have served so many not only afflicted in the body but in the mind and the soul and again reaffirming *Pranprathisthan* within, I request Swamiji to feel so cool, so very cool as we are really, we are in some Antarctic region. It's getting cool, cooler. Yes and so much cooler but all the time comfortable. In this experience of cooler and cooler, in the perfect trance of meditative way we are translocated. Yes the several locations at times Narmada flows wide and at other times we see the turbulent waters of Narmada going around Jabalpur and the magnificent town of Indore and holiest all places. Holiest of the holiest places where Ganges has washed away through the millennium the *kleshas* of millions and millions of people. Quiet flows the Ganga in Banaras and the dark deep mystic Yamuna flows across Delhi and somehow somewhere Ganga and Kaveri are one. And Swami Vivekananada said and he said to us that the rivers flow and flow in these all different ways, Sindhu, Ganga, Yamuna, Narmada, Tapi, Kaveri, Krishna and the Adyar river in Chennai they all flow with mystic light and Swami Vivekananda said through their different parts they all merge into ocean. As your right hand has moved we have seen the ocean where all the rivers of the world have merged themselves into an eternity and we are watching that cool (3) and very, very cold ocean of Antartica. I feel the coolness around you and your right hand is cool, your left hand is cool.

You have let gone all the heat that generates tension.

Swamiji's heart has always been cool, all cool, cool, all over the body and in the Antarctic Ocean. The freezing beauty of the snow, the magnificent light of the midnight sun, Swamiji sees the sun of the *Brahmamuhurta*[20], right before his eyes and that as well is the sun of midnight in this Antartica region.

And Swamiji is pondering. Swamiji is pondering over the wonders of so many icebergs and Swamiji is counting the icebergs before his eyes. 1, 2, 3 and Swamiji will count as many icebergs that he sees. And in counting of the icebergs as the counting goes all the heat of the accumulated *kleshas* withers; and breathe, let them so relaxed, let the pleasant, beneficient, benevolent mind, of Swamiji's childlike face beam all across.

1/9th of the iceberg, i.e. 1, 2, 3, 4 as many as you have counted Swamiji but you will work with the iceberg of your choice, the iceberg or all the icebergs that Swamiji is capable of handling, any and as many as all of them, or all at once or one by one or the only one that Swamiji has chosen to do. When you have decided to begin with the iceberg, Swamiji yes your natural due to so perfectly.

Relax, Swamiji that you might be in transcendental sleep, where there is a transcendental awakening in the transcendental sleep also. When you have made up your mind to deal with the iceberg or all the icebergs, kindly let me know by the movement of any of your fingers of the right hand. Swamiji is tackling the iceberg of his choice, iceberg of his choice reveals only 1/9th of the tip and is so cool, so deep as Swamiji has put both his hands within the ice of the ice cube that Swamiji's hands are getting cold, cold and colder and so much colder that they are like frozen ice. Swamiji's hands are ice cold. There is a numbness, numbness, tingling is also going away, the touch has also disappeared, the sense of touch is gone, the sense of frozenness in the left hand has set in, and the work is going on, and the work is going on with both the hands. Your left hand is totally cold. How nice to work with the iceberg and Swamiji's hands are extremely deeper and deeper into the iceberg.

And it is your choice Swamiji, how much you want to dip into the iceberg. And as you have continued with the iceberg, your left hand is totally devoid of all sensations as I pass my hand over your left hand, over your left hand. It is totally numb, totally numb and painless. Relax yourself Swamiji, there is a slight hypodermic prick and in that slight hypodermic prick, there is a deep deep breath,

Swamiji continue to work with that iceberg, deep deep breath, the left hand is now feeling no more pain.

As is your right hand totally numb, totally numb, so much so numb, entirely without any sensation, so much so that the left hand has the slight of the slightest sensation. When your right hand has become numb, you are working with us, right hand is freezing, much more freezing, frozen then left and so frozen that when you want to move your fingers you are unable to move them. Deep, deep and deeper breath, deeper and deeper state of trance, higher and higher state of *Annamaya, Pranamaya, Manomaya, Vijnanamaya,* and *Anandamaya Koshas*[21], Swamiji, entirely and completely established in *Anandmaya Kosha*, your right hand is frozen. You are unable to move any of your fingers. Try to move any of your fingers, Swamiji, you are not able to move any of the fingers of the right hand because they are frozen. Wonderful How Very Wonderful, Most Wonderful. Now you are coming out of the trance as I start counting from 10 to 1. 10..9..8..7..6..5..4..3..2..1.. Now that you have come out of the trance, try and move your hand at the level of the shoulder. See whether you are feeling the pain that you had. You are completely awake and painfree. Congratulations, you have made it.

Now your hand is coming back to normal temperature with your left hand you are feeling the touch. Sensations are back but pain is gone for good. Out of sight, out of mind, never to come again. All work is a worship.

The frozen shoulder was made to feel pain free by a pin prick. When he was pain free, gradually the coolness was brought to normal temperature and he felt his pain free condition. Gradually he got the sensation of touch back without pain. His movements of the shoulder were normal. We met him after 5 years and said he is completely pain free.

Case 2 : A lady doctor who was a Christian nun, complained of allergy to soaps. She tried various kinds of soaps for body and washing the clothes. After giving her a session, she was cured.

Next day when she reported, she said 'I tried all soaps to what I was allergic, I can use all of them'.

The same way as the previous case, she also was a medical doctor and was reassigned to a table job of administration from her regular medical practice. She was put into the deep trance. The suggestion revolved around 'only thing permanent is change'.

The two cases that we have discussed required a regular induction of trance by hypnotherapy. While Maharshi like Sri Aurobindo and Raman Maharshi, tolerated the pain of fracture and surgery with their experience of *Samadhi*[22], this would always be a point of discussion. It will require hypnotherapist's acumen to judge whether the subject would require induction and deepening!!!

Gene Expression Studies

Ernest Rossi has exhorted us that we should study the gene expression following hypnotherapy since that would prove his highly publicized hypothesis. We applied for a 6 cr. grant in collaboration with Prof. Nagaraja, at NIMHANS. The story of his failure is narrated elsewhere. However, we persisted with our efforts with some money that was raised at 2009 national conference.

Melatonin is a hormone secreted by the pineal gland. It needs expression of only two genes. Therefore, the study of only two genes that would be minimally expensive and yet be an indirect proof that early expression genes are activated with long term usage of therapy. When an experiment conducted at M.S. University with deeply hypnotized subjects did not reveal any higher levels of melatonin[23], Avnish Dave persisted with practitioners of long term meditation. Meditation is equated to self hypnosis, this study is also proving that a long term hypnotherapeutic application may also see the high levels of melatonin.

Avnish Dave has added one more dimension to contemporization. This is derived from ancient Tantric practice; yet the relevance is evident since there is sound anatomical basis. Autonomic nervous system is silently regulated by balancing between sympathetic and parasympathetic systems. There is high connectivity between the nerve plexuses. Two systems have profound interconnectivity at some of the regions. Avnish Dave targets the plexuses at various levels, beginning from sacral region to the cerebrum.

There are 7 *chakras* in the body. *Muladhar chakra* is based at the pelvis in the coxygial region. The second one is the *Svadhisthana chakra* located in the hypogastrium. The third, *Manipur chakra* is located at the solar plexus. The next is *Anahat chakra* which is located in the region of the heart. The *Vishuddha chakra* is located in the throat region of thyroid. *Ajna chakra*, located in the forehead, between the 2 eyebrows. Lastly, the *Sahasrar chakra* located in the brain, right and left hemisphere have tremendous connectivity via corpus callosum though the hemispheres differ to some extent in their function, whole brain functioning is established via corpus callosum.

Interconnectivity between sympathetic and parasympathetic systems as well as their anatomical continuity has provided hypnotherapists to focus on their stimulation for an energy depleted person.

There cannot be a final closure without inclusion of *Bhagavad Gita:* a holy book for all Hindus. However, its secular appeal is across religions. In Germany, Friedrich Max Muller and in recent times, Andreas Reimers, a neurologist with his M.D. thesis based on transcendental meditation and Romain Rolland have been inspired from the teachings of the *Bhagavad Gita*. Even during the Iron curtain era of Stalin rule, Alexander Solzhenitsyn, a Nobel laureate, in his novel depicted the hero deriving solace from *Bhagavad Gita* when deported to Siberia. *Mahabhạrata* as a long epic, has several archetypal symbols but to the uninitiated even, *Bhagavad Gita* can help as a hypnotherapeutic manual for application to several psychiatric disorders.

Therefore, we have included an entire chapter by Dr. Dipankar Patra.

Notes

1. Stone guardians at the gates of a temple.
2. Golden crown.
3. One of Devi Durga's forms as killer of demon Mahishasur.
4. Slowly.
5. Quiet.
6. Steady.
7. Without worry.
8. Carefree.
9. True or eternal self.
10. Illusion.
11. Devotional hymn to Hanuman.
12. A melodic mode or structure in Indian Classical Music.
13. Philosopher.
14. Divine Bliss descending from above (*Bhagavad Gita* 18-14).
15. Invoke deity.
16. 4th state of consciousness.
17. Disturbances or conflicts in mind.
18. Poor soul.
19. State of being free from mental distress.
20. 48-minute period (*muhurta*) that begins one hour and 36 minutes before sunrise, and ends 48 minutes before sunrise.
21. *Koshas* are sheaths of energy that are defined as *Annamaya*—Nutrition, *Pranmaya*—Vitality, *Manomaya*—Mind, *Vijnanmaya*—Intellect, *Anandmaya*—Bliss.
22. 7th state of consciousness.
23. Assessment of melatonin levels in normal healthy young university students, post hypnosis and yoga practitioners, Avnish D., Jayant M., *et al.*; *International Journal of Basic and Applied Physiology*, *8*(1), 2019 pp. 82-85.

4

Metaphors in *Bhagavad Gita* and *Bhagavad Gita* as a Metaphor*

Hypnosis and hypnotherapy have been in vogue from time immemorial in India. They are closer to the Indian psyche in terms of format and treatment. In this chapter, hypnotherapy is discussed in the Indian context with its socio-cultural and spiritual perspectives. Although there are hundreds of scriptures in our *Santana parampara*[1], the study is based primarily on *Gita.* Certain concepts, like *Maya, Samatvam*[2], *Manoshuddhi*[3], *Viyoga*[4], *Advaita*[5], *Viveka*[6], *Shama*[7], *Vaktapas*[8], *Atmabodh*[9], and *Moksha*[10] from the Indian *shastras*[11] have been referenced to hypnosis, especially in relation to Ericksonian hypnotherapy. Various stages of hypnotherapy from trance induction to trance termination and post-hypnotic suggestion have been studied in relation to concepts from *Sanatana Dharma.*[12] The qualities of a hypnotherapist have also been highlighted. The author who has been a practicing hypnotherapist for over 2 decades feels that it is very essential for all hypnotherapists practicing in India to have a proper understanding and assimilation of the phenomenological,

*Dipankar Patra Ph.D, Vice President, Indian Society for Clinical & Experimental Hypnosis.

ontological, and spiritual synthesis of this wonderful subject to derive the utmost therapeutic benefits.

Keywords: Hypnosis, hypnotherapy, suggestion, trance.

Introduction

Case study: Profile of the client: On a winter night, I received a frantic call from an unknown number. This man, probably in his late 30s, a bystander, discovered a septuagenarian, who was walking aimlessly towards the Metro railway tracks of a nearby station. Fearing that the aged man was trying to put an end to his life, the young man accosted the old man who did not reveal anything to him initially but when threatened to inform the police, took out from his pocket what appeared to be my visiting card. In the next half an hour I was talking to this old patient of mine who had come to me some weeks back for depression-related issues after he lost his wife to Covid. Prof Amlan Sen (name changed) was an ex-professor of Psychology at a reputed college in Kolkata. I remember him as a person who was well-read in our *Shastras* and who took pride in our rich culture and heritage.

Prof Amlan seemed to have lots of dreams about his son who had changed for the worse, especially after his marriage. He narrated how his son and daughter-in-law forcefully evicted him from his ancestral home and admitted him to an Old age Home. They had managed to transfer his ancestral property in their name and he did not seem to have any place in their busy lives. Loneliness, alienation, and politically disillusioned, he was having a problem finding meaning and sense in continuing with a seemingly purposeless life and had recurrent suicidal ideation too.

He had been to a psychiatrist but the medicines did not ease his problems. While recuperating at a hospital for a fortnight, he had as a company, a Bengali version of the *Bhagavad Gita* (BG) which surprisingly gave him some solace and served him as a survival guide. The helplessness, feeling of being alienated, and extreme anxiety were too much for him to bear and he was caught in a conflict of fighting for his rights or accepting this destiny with a calm, resigned, and stoic acceptance.

While I was talking to him, I realized that I could utilize the Ericksonian principle of Observation and Utilization to deal with his situation. Borrowing examples and allusions from the *Bhagavad Gita* itself, we could instill a sense of despondency and urgency to deal with the right *Dharmic*[13] conflicts for him. We had the most profound of discussions, the most intense of therapy at the most unusual of places—on the streets of a quiet Kolkata night.

Although a Psychologist he was not much aware of hypnosis and like most people had some myths to be dispelled. However, he was an enthusiast, a quick learner, and had no qualms about sharing and receiving knowledge. When he wanted to find out whether hypnotherapy could actually help someone similar to his kind of distress, I realized that I had a crucial and meaningful role to play.

In this document, as far as practicable there has been a deliberate usage of Sanskrit words like *Dhyana*, *shastra*, *vasanas*, and *sanskars* instead of the wrongly attributed words like meditation, scriptures, desires, and cultures, respectively as the latter miss out the very essence of the Indian ethos and culture which is essentially spiritual. The purpose of the document is to develop a sense of pride, relatedness, and ownership of all hypnotherapists practicing in India so that one can understand the multidimensional nature of the subject.

Following are the excerpts from our discussion based on the Professor's queries and his first query centred around various topics surrounding hypnosis, the first being my vocation as a hypnotherapist.

The role of a hypnotherapist: In a psychotherapeutic context, the capability to understand the mind of the subject is central to a hypnotherapist and the essence of finding relief in therapy starts with choosing the right hypnotherapist having the requisite attitude, knowledge, and skills for therapeutic healing. As is reflected and repeated in *Gita*, the client needs to be able to have humility and total surrender.

***Overcome by anxiety and weakness, I am confused about my duties. I surrender to You as Your disciple. Please instruct me in my best interest.* (*B.G., 2.7*)**

Along with the attitude of total submission, one also needs to repose totality in trust and *shraddha.*[14]

***Leave everything and Trust me, I will rescue you from all the problems, do not worry.* (*B.G., 18.66*).**

One of the causes of the superior therapeutic efficacy of hypnotherapy is the establishment of a strong rapport or a "communion in consciousness" (Vyas & Vyas, 2009). Krishna, the therapist, cautions that therapy is to be provided to only the one who seeks it intently and the client should voluntarily seek help. Although, unless there is a Karmic communion there can be no communion between the *Guru* and *shishya*[15] therapist and the client, knowledge and therapy should be judiciously applied by the therapist to only the needy and deserving. In the *Bhagavad Gita*, Krishna says:

***This confidential knowledge may never be explained to those who are not austere, devoted, or engaged in devotional service (seva), nor to one who is envious of Me.* (*B.G., 18.67*)**

Easwaran (1997) notes that in the Hindu tradition, until we ask the teacher to be our *guru*, showing our readiness to receive his guidance on the path of *dhyana*, he does not offer to do this for us. Also, it is the wise who can seek help as they insist upon not deluding the minds of those who are not ready, unprepared, or unwilling for counselling and psychotherapy (***na buddhi bhedam janayeda jnanam karma sanginam***) and in truth, the efficacy of a true and successful therapy and the skills of the psychotherapist spreads more effectively when shared by word of mouth.

***But sharing this topmost secret qualifies as the highest form of work in devotion and such a devotee will surely come back to Me.* (*B.G., 18.68*)**

The hypnotherapist utilizes his intuitive understanding more effectively to understand the client. Intuition is a faculty that can be cultivated through long association of studying scriptures or spiritual *sadhana.*[16] Through the client and therapy, the therapist develops a transcendental intuitive knowledge about a deeper and sublime meaning of life. This understanding is intuitive and beyond the realms of the five senses and the mind.

Along with intuition, insightful sensory understanding is of paramount importance in hypnotherapy. To become a good hypnotherapist, one needs to be knowledgeable in various disciplines and have multiple strategies in his armoury. Thus, intuition and insight along with *swaadhyaya*[17] or guidance under a *guru* are very essential for one's spiritual growth and Krishna recommends the *Shastras* to be the manual for the psychoeducation of people in distress.

Let the Shastras be your authority in determining what should be done and what should not be done. Understand the scriptural injunctions and teachings, and then perform your actions in this world accordingly. (B.G., 16.24)

But all knowledge is incomplete and ineffective without the judicious application of principles, techniques, and patterns, best exemplified in the workings of Milton Erickson and much later by Stephen Brooks, the pioneer of Compassionate Ericksonian hypnotherapy. Thus, the scriptures contain observations of those who have walked along the spiritual path but mere observation has no value whatsoever if there are no practical therapeutic applications of it.

In chapter 16 of *The Gita*, Krishna highlights the potentialities or qualities (*gunas*) of a happy man, most of which are in essence a prerequisite of a hypnotherapist. They are: fearlessness (*abhyam*), purity of heart (*sattva samshuddhi*), almsgiving (*dana*), self-restraint (*dama*), right study of the *Shastras* (*svadhyaya*), self-discipline (*tapas)*, straightforwardness (*arjavam*), non-injury (*ahimsa*), truth (*satya*), absence of wrath (*akrodha*), peace (*shanti)*, absence of fault finding and calumny (*apaishunam)*, compassion towards all things (*daya)*, non-covetousness, absence of greed (*aloluptvam*), modesty (*hri*), patience or fortitude (*dhriti*), purity of body and mind (*shaucha*), non-hatred (*aduesha*), lack of conceit (*na atimanita*), amongst others.

Meditation/Hypnotherapy is essentially therapeutic spiritual. Swami Sivananda in *Sadhana Chatustaya* mentions about 4 spiritual qualities as per *Vedic* knowledge, which the Vedantins believe will lead to *Brahma Gyan* or transcendental knowledge. They are *Viveka* (spiritual discernment), *Vairagyam* (Non-attachment), *Mumukshutvam* (intense earning for self-realization), and *Shadsampat* (6 cognitive virtues: thought control, sense control, lifestyle stability, forbearance, *shraddha*, and inner tranquility). They are essentially a sequence of steps or means of practice that are outlined in the teachings of *Vedanta* and *Jnana Yoga* which is essential for hypnotherapists. They must be cultivated on the path to self-realization, and form the foundation for deeper therapeutic understanding and development.

Having understood the qualities of a hypnotherapist, Prof Amlan Sen then wanted to understand hypnosis and its relation to Indian psychotherapy.

Indic origins of Hypnosis: Our great spiritual *gurus* have considered that mankind is in a sort of hypnotic trance, hypnotized by situations, attractions from the external material world, and beliefs, and that to wake up from it and make the mind multidimensional it is essential to de-hypnotize oneself.

Hypnosis (Greek '*Hypnos*') originally meant sleep and is probably attributed to the practice of Greeks and Romans performing rituals concerning death and rebirth called, "Temples of Sleep". In India, however, the practice of taking the sick to the local temple to get treated has existed since time immemorial. There can be no wonder that the state of hypnosis was known to Indian sages from antiquity, much before what is commonly attributed to the Greeks or Europeans, like Anton Mesmer, James Braid, James Esdaile, and others. This is also corroborated by the account of the famous historian, Durant (1937). Vyas & Vyas (2017) mentioned that Patanjali's *Yoga Sutra* was a road map to *dhyana* and hypnotic skills that are generated automatically within the practitioner. The subject of hypnosis and the practice of hypnotherapy have always been present in India since the *Vedic* times, which was essentially therapeutic and spiritual in content and form. Unfortunately, due to our colonial hangover, we still have a lot of internal and external resistance to relate this to our golden lineage.

Avasthi, Kate, and Grover (2013), rightly state that people practicing psychotherapy in India generally have a myopic approach that largely ignores the multi-diversity of cultures, languages, ethnicity, religious affiliations, the role of family, eastern philosophy, and holistic treatment in understanding and managing problems. Bhawuk (2011) noted that in the past few decades, in India, "psychology moved away from its Indian roots to mimic Western method and theory". The Western approach did not appear to fit to the Indian psyche and anything that did not fit the Western model was considered an anomaly". However, it is heart rendering to understand that in recent times there has been a greater emphasis on subjective experience and a person-centric approach, and psychology and psychotherapy are gradually moving towards a consciousness-based approach, the roots of which are in our *Shastras.* Psychotherapy and especially, hypnotherapy is gradually becoming short-termed, crisis-oriented, supportive, flexible, eclectic, and spiritual.

An understanding of concepts borrowed from our *Shastras* is very essential for psychotherapeutic practice. Anecdotes from the Indian *Shastras,* and mythological texts contain transcendental therapeutic wisdom which helps to explain better psychiatric symptoms, psychological principles, unconscious conflicts, defense mechanisms, automatic thoughts and cognitive errors. Added to this, the philosophical belief of the transmigration of the soul, rebirth, fatalism, the different nature and quantum of guilt feeling, and the difference in the expectation as well as the environment manipulation are some of the glaring differences a therapist working in India should prioritize.

Manusmriti (the famous ancient *Shastra*s of the Indian sage Manu) categorizes hypnosis into different stages and based on its effect, hypnosis has the "Sleep-Waking" state, the "Dream-Sleep" state, and the "Ecstasy-Sleep" state. However, the earliest reference to hypnosis is probably the *Atharva Veda* which mentioned *Mantra Vidya* as the main technique for *manas chikitsa* or the treatment of the mind. *Mantra vidya* relied heavily on the meaning and vibration of sounds and was used in 5 types of therapies of which *Sankalpa* (auto suggestion), *Sandesha* (suggestions by the therapist) and *Samavashikarana* (application of hypnosis) are relevant to modern-day hypnosis. Max-Muller and Bloomfield (1897) mention the reference to hypnosis and suggestion in *Atharvaveda* (4:13:7): "Touching you with these two hands and ten fingers, by my influential speech I speak to you, disease removing words. By this, you will get healthy and all your diseases will vanish."

We also come across the concept of *siddhis* in *Vibhuti pada* of sage Patanjali's *Yoga Sutras* which include *vashita,* which is the ability to control the will of others. The concept of control, however, was essentially for therapeutic healing and did not imply any form of coercion. References to hypnosis can also be found in Vagbhatta's *Ashtanga Samhita* which deals with the treatment of various forms of psychosomatic disorders. According to Abhay Charan De, later popularly known as Swami Prabhupada (1955), the *Bhagwat Purana* has evidence of the use of *sammohanavidya* where Lord Vishnu in his *Mohini avatar* alludes to the *asuras* (demons) to procure the *Amrit Kumbha* for the *devas* (gods). This *Sammohana,* which was "a state of inner balance that radiates positivity around, influencing, and enchanting others" (Malhotra & Babaji, 2021) was prevalent since the *Vedic* times. It was generally practiced by people who were balanced and centred inside and who radiated a positive charismatic aura around themselves.

***Dhyana* and hypnotherapy:** The word *dhyana,* derived from the root *dhyai* in Sanskrit means to think or contemplate and encompasses a much deeper connotation than the reductionist, over-simplified, and widely used term meditation. While *Dhyana* is a specific limb of *Ashtanga Yoga* revealed by Sage Patanjali, the term meditation is used indiscriminately to denote the latter 5 limbs of *yoga*, collapsing many technical aspects of the *sadhana* into one ill-defined word. Historically and pragmatically distinct, hypnosis and *dhyana* share much in the way of phenomenology, neurocognitive mechanisms, and potential therapeutic prospects. Techniques of *Dhyana* are similar to hypnosis and while the path is the same, the direction is different.

In their work, Patra, D. & Neelakandan, R. (2021) emphasize the fact that the approach of hypnosis, being close to Indian *Yoga* and meditative *sadhana* is "suited to the Indian psyche, and works as an integrative and holistic treatment". Indians believe hypnosis has its roots in ancient *Yoga Nidra* (or Yogic sleep) which is indiscriminately spiritual. *Yoga Nidra* involves concepts of *pratyahara* (inward withdrawal of senses), *dharana* (engaging the mind on a particular area), and *dhyana* (mind flowing in an unbroken current towards a particular point), from Patanjali's *Yoga Sutra*s. They also included other concepts like *Shavasana* and muscular relaxation. Very recently, the term *Yoga Nidra* is popularised by Swami Satyananda Saraswati (1976) of Bihar School of Yoga, which centres around the practice, which is very similar to hypnosis.

Learnings from *The Gita* about hypnotherapy: *The Gita* along with the *Upanishads* and the *Brahma Sutra* form a part of *Prasthan Trayi* (scriptural trinity) and according to Rao (1980), it is based partly on *Ishavashya upanishad* and *Kathopanishad.* Scholars have identified various therapeutic components in *The Gita* which are also prevalent in other Indian *Shastras.* There are elements of *Samkhya Yoga*—relating to maladaptive cognition, *Karma Yoga*—relating to work with an attitude of renunciation, *Gyan Karma Sannyasa Yoga*—Intelligent approach to work without any form of anxiety, *Gyan Vigyan Yoga*—insight-oriented learnings, *Bhakti Yoga*—therapy based on love, compassion, and total surrender. *The Gita* also contains other psychological techniques, such as Behaviour therapy, like, flooding—involving prolonged and continuous exposure to anxiety-provoking situations on the battlefield itself; Catharsis or ventilation, and finally, Cognitive hypnotherapy. In the *Bhagavad Gita*, Krishna addressed the cognitive and emotional issues of Arjuna, who is representative of the entire mankind. He leads him from the transitory to the eternal, from a false understanding of the ego to go beyond suffering. Like a cognitive hypnotherapist who corrects the cognitive error of the client through a dialectic process involving thought, action, feeling, and behaviour. Krishna leads Arjuna to a deeper understanding of the self and actions.

From a psychotherapeutic perspective, Arjuna is the client or subject and, Krishna is the hypnotherapist. Their relationship is closer to a *Guru-Shishya* relationship (Reddy, 2012). One of the names of Krishna is *Mohana,* which means the one who enchants or hypnotizes. Swami Prabhupada (1999) refers to the enchanting tunes Krishna used to play on his flute for the *gopis* in Vrindavan who were simply mesmerized. Technically, the entire *Gita* is a single-session therapy where the therapist stays with the client throughout the therapy. The Kurukshetra war from a psychological point of view, represents a fundamental transformation in the psychological life of man, and in the end, the ultimate discovery is that the psychological problem resides neither in the object nor in the senses—it abides in the mind, which needs to be surmounted.

Mehta (1995) contends that the *Gita* indicates a way of life that is intensely revolutionary, for it speaks not merely of an extension of consciousness but most assuredly of an expansion of it. He asserts that the journey of the *Gita* is from Mind to super Mind, and from Intellect to Intuition. While Arjuna stands for the mind, alert and active, Krishna symbolizes the Super Mind. Thus, the *Gita* is a book of spiritual revolution and not of a mere social or behavioural reformation. It is a path toward divinity. Hypnosis is a platform that helps to give one this taste of divinity.

Hypnosis is all about intuition and dealing with the unconscious. The teachings of *The Gita* abound in the role of the unconscious in the form of *samskaras* or acts done to purify the existence of a person and make one's body worthy of the *atman*. These acts or habits are the preceptors of human behaviour and often these *samskaras* come from our past impressions.

Ericksonian hypnotherapy: Stories of immense possibility: Ericksonian approach to hypnotherapy uses stories, fables and parables, allusions, metaphors, similes, etc. to elucidate understanding which can be aimed at addressing different levels of one's transformational journey. They are trance-inducing and insightfully therapeutic. There is a very interesting story of a father and son described in the *Chandogya Upanishad* that highlights the immense potential, as humans we carry within us. The father asks the son to peel off a seed progressively and the son discovers that in the end there is nothing left. It is wonderful to know that the whole tree grows from the nothingness of the seed and that the Self resides inside the seed, from which this enormous tree has sprung forth. We forget our infinite presence and unlimited potential and are often caught fretting over the finite and trivial. Thus, the meaning of existence is to be found in Non-existence—the significance of all things lies in No-things. This knowledge is existential and is submerged deep within us and hypnosis and *Dhyana* are tools to unravel and discover deep-rooted hidden potentials of an individual by accessing the unconscious. In hypnosis, one also discovers intuitively that one is the *Ananda* (happiness) one seeks and that this state of happiness reflects our inner calling which is related to our *svabhava* and *svadharma* (Being and Becoming).

"***The wise person must live in accordance with their unique inner calling, or dharma***". **(*B.G., 3.35*)**

It is this unique inner calling that is essential to one's spiritual journey and the role of a hypnotherapist is to trigger the latent possibilities of an individual by accessing the deepest recesses of the mind.

We also discussed some concepts from the Shastras relevant to hypnotherapy.

Understanding the concept of *Maya:* *Maya* is spiritual in essence and denotes the creative *Shakti* of *Brahman* or *Bhagavan.* Its function is to conceal the truth and to project something false in the place of truth. It casts a hypnotic spell on us, strikes universally, and almost "bewitches" our minds.

"Souls' wisdom is veiled by ignorance. Hence human beings are deluded." (B.G., 5.15)

Swami Vivekananda (1947) in discourse with his Western audience felt that in this material world, we are already hypnotized and that *Vedanta* can help us to de-hypnotize. He said, "Hindus, de-hypnotize yourselves. Let us proclaim to every soul: Arise, awake, and do not stop until the goal is attained.

Sri Paramhansa Yogananda (2002) refers to the verses in *The Gita* from verse 7.13 to 7.20—describing *Viswarup darshan*—as a state of "cosmic hypnosis" and suggests ways to transcend it. He mentions that like a person in a dreaming state cannot capture the consciousness of his waking state, worldly men are in a state of "cosmic dream delusion which is imposed like a hypnotic spell on men from birth and they remain unaware of its insidiousness." He suggests we need to de-hypnotize from cosmic delusion by surrendering to the supreme hypnotherapist, Krishna.

As hypnosis is a powerful tool to access the deepest layers of an individual, it aids in removing delusions by including an experiential discourse at a deeper unconscious level. This ensures one has a transcendental knowledge that frees one from the spell of disempowering *Maya* and contributes to the disappearance of *avidya* (false knowledge and delusion).

Developing *Samatvam* (Emotional equanimity): *Samatvam* relates to an insightful understanding of one's inner resources during therapy and a hypnotherapist needs to develop such qualities.

For one who has mastered their mind and who is tranquil, the supreme Self is self-evident. (The knower of Self remains the same in heat and cold, pleasure and pain, joy and sorrow as well as in honour and infamy. (B.G., 6.7)

Emotional equanimity can be achieved by living in total awareness and through the practice of *abhyasena* (self-effort) and *vairagyam* (detachment). One signifies action, the other inaction (*B.G., 6.35*).

Ensuring Mental purification (*Manoshuddhi*): Mental purification involves identifying our thoughts, beliefs, and concepts. Our life and our character become what we believe (*yad bhavam tad bhawati*). Sleepwalking and mass hypnosis continue feeding the fire of our voracious delusions and the only way out of it is through *dhyana* and hypnosis. Thus, a hypnotherapist needs to develop an unalloyed nature of thoughts and behaviour that utilizes the components of sensory perception, emotional involvement, the cognitive factor, and of course, the spiritual component.

***Viyoga*: Cultivating detachment from possession and people:** Attachment alone is the main cause of unhappiness and the only we to go beyond is to be able to discriminate between healthy and unhealthy desires.

***O scion of Bharata, the ignorant act attached to the results of their action whilst the wise act without those attachments, thereby inspiring the masses.* (*B.G., 3.25*)**

The *Gita* explains the cycle of *samsara* and suffering in detail. Thus, the first stage of attachment (*abhilasa*) is desire, consisting of attachment (*raga*) and aversion (*dwesha*). Unfulfilled desire is transformed into grief, anxiety, self-pity (*shoka*), and then anger (*krodha*). Anger leads to temporary insanity called delusion (*moha*) and in this stage one is in a stage of spiritual forgetfulness (*smriti-nasha)* or corrupted wisdom (*buddhi nasha*).This understanding is the foundation of all forms of psychotherapy and remaining unattached is the hallmark of happiness.

A cognitive hypnotherapist helps in cultivating and practicing controlled detachment (*viyoga*) from possession and people by cutting the ropes of attachment and reclaiming one's inner freedom, therapeutically. The therapist needs to first understand the type of attachment that leads to one's suffering and then help one to get rid of the *samsara* by cultivating awareness, during trance.

Development of the concept of *Advaita* (Non-dualism): The cultivation of a sense of non-duality or Oneness which is the essence of *Vedanta* helps one to transcend the ego and develop a strong sense of emotional maturity and a state of eternal *Ananda.* The main obstacles in the path of non-duality are our *vasanas,* which are innate psychological urges or subconscious pre-dispositions of desires.

Hypnotherapy also helps one to experientially enjoy this state of non-duality by helping one by transcending the false ego and to access these maladaptive deliberations and move to an enlightened realization.

Understanding of the concept of *Nitya-Anitya* (Permanence-Impermanence): Finding this sense of unity in all existence follows from a deeper understanding of the impermanent nature of our being. Thus, acceptance of both misery and happiness, permanence and impermanence aspects of our being through an elevated profound vision of an eternal reality is the first step towards the development of higher and profound wisdom. Hypnosis is one of the powerful tools to access such wisdom. Perfect healing or psychotherapeutic intervention can only happen if a good hypnotherapist awakens spiritually because only then one can cultivate sense of acceptance and compassion and move beyond the permanence and impermanence nature of existence.

Cultivating *Bhawashuddhi* (Emotional intelligence): Emotional maturity rests in one by having the right control of thoughts and emotions, as reflected in *The Gita.*

Absolute freedom exists on all sides for the self-controlled ones who are free from cravings and anger, who have controlled their thoughts and have therefore realized the Self. (B.G., 5.26)

To be aware of the functioning of the *tamas,* the *rajas,* and the *sattva* and yet not interfere with them is to be free from all conditioning. It is essential for a hypnotherapist to understand the personality type of an individual based on the *gunas* before designing the route for therapy. Once the emotion is identified and classified, the hypnotherapist then attempts to diffuse negative emotions in a sequence. As he understands that only a change in thoughts can lead to a change in feelings. Then, in a therapeutic environment, the hypnotherapist guides one's resolve not to suppress emotions but identifies the source of the intense emotions, and helps make one accept their vulnerability and self-ignorance by practicing forgiveness and cultivating self-love.

Experiencing inner witness (*Sakshi*): The outcome of the feeling of dispassionate dissociation as a result of being a witness is central to any form of therapeutic healing. To be a witness implies that one is watching and observing objectively, without identifying oneself with the object of observation. Witnessing consciousness is a powerful *sadhana* as evidenced in the *Mandukya Upanishad.* Developing the right *sakshibhav* helps one to remain detached from one's thoughts, beliefs, and perceptions. The most significant experience during hypnosis is being able to transcend the limited ego self and being a pure witness. Powerful techniques like age regression, age vivification, and visualization techniques involving multiple mirror exercises help one to drop all identity and become a pure objective witness, during hypnotherapy.

Moving towards V*airagyam* (humility): Humility is transcending the ego state of an individual and grace is bestowed on anyone showing humility and compassion. It is a quality worth emulating by hypnotherapists and it is the foundation of one's spiritual growth and the experience of hypnosis ensures one's experiential understanding of it. Once a hypnotherapist can cultivate humility, he can also practice gratitude and forgiveness, two essential qualities of a healer and a therapist.

Practicing *Viveka* (Discrimination) and Hypnosis: The practice of *Viveka* or discernment involves moment-by-moment deliberation before acting or reacting. Our *Shastras* highlight that the prerequisite to cultivating *Viveka* is to be able to distinguish the quality of mental experience of a person observed through the 3 qualities or *gunas*—*sattva* (illuminating *guna*), *rajas* (a*Gita*ting *guna*), and *tamas* (dulling *guna*). The knowledge enshrined in the *Upanishads* and *The Gita* speaks of the 3 *gunas* which are very essential for a hypnotherapist to understand and apply in a therapeutic context.

The hypnotherapist instills an intuitive understanding in the client that the means of escape from misery is constant discrimination that starts with monitoring of an emotional experience. He understands that each individual is unique and hence the prognosis and the treatment should also lend subjectivity. Hypnotherapy is aimed at therapeutically building a *Sattvic* mind of an individual by helping one to find their resources of being: focused, discerning, decisive, mature, steady, expansive, unadulterated, subtle, sharp & spiritual. All this starts with effective thought management.

Imbibing *Shama* (thoughts management): *Shama* is the foundation of Cognitive hypnotherapy. A hypnotherapist helps one to learn cognitive skills like thought management and the science of ethics. First, intellectually, then emotionally, one is led to the perception of unity over diversity. In an individual, the concept of bondage and freedom, power and powerlessness, all occur in the realm of the thought, and in hypnotherapy, one can be led to transcend beyond these realms.

One should uplift oneself by one's efforts: One should not lower oneself. For the purified mind alone is the friend of oneself: the non-purified mind alone is the enemy of oneself. (B.G., 6.5).

One of the powerful tools of cognitive thought management is *Pratipaksha Bhavan* or a method of deliberately thinking of the opposites. This is also foundational to the subject of Neuroplasticity. In hypnosis, the hypnotherapist sometimes deliberately guides an aggrieved person to conceive of something opposite, constructive, and dharmic so that the mind of the sufferer expands from delusion to clarity, from selfishness to selflessness, from material to spiritual and this change happens unconsciously, which is more experiential than cognitive. One's conscious mind is deliberately distracted, confused, or overloaded with ambiguous language. Confusion techniques to prevent it from analyzing, the therapist's suggestions and controlling unconscious responses, a practice widely used by Ericksonian hypnotherapists.

Our *Shastras* abound with *shlokas*, *sutras*, and *mantras* which appear to be apparently contradictory at the superficial level but intelligibly designed to cater to the spiritual seeker for having a deeper, intuitive understanding. A client or a patient subjected to such deliberate confusion has no other option but to dive deep within oneself to fathom the seeming contradiction and find answers. An example of confusion is when Krishna narrates: ***Amongst cheaters, I am a gambler.* (*B.G., 10.36*)**

Finally, one of the chief ways one can practice *Shama* is through having control of speech and silence.

***Vaaktapas* (communication protocols) and hypnotherapy:** The *Gita* mentions non-violent speech (*anudvegkaramvaak*), truthful speech (*satyamvaak*), pleasant speech (*priyamvaak*), and beneficial speech (*hitamvaak*) and Krishna also speaks of silence with reference to the mind and not with reference to speech.

***Non-violent speech, which is truthful, pleasant, and beneficial and used to utter the Vedic truth is called austerity of speech.* (*B.G., 17.15*)**

A hypnotherapist has to utilize the right kind of speech and also silence both during trance induction and therapy by carefully observing and analyzing the client's verbal and non-verbal language. He needs to first embody inner silence within himself to support conscious speech. Indeed, pauses between hypnotic suggestions can be very effective in both trance induction and therapy, and with practice when silence compliments mindful speech, the inner tranquillity in a hypnotherapist increases manyfold and he becomes an empathetic listener, as well.

The ultimate takeaways in hypnosis: *Atmabodha* and *Moksha*: In the Indian tradition, *Moksha* is believed to be the ultimate end of a spiritual journey. *Moksha* (Sanskrit *muchyate*) means free or released from the bondage of *samsara* and is the ultimate solution for-end-of world distress. It is a permanent experience and this awakening does not fluctuate. It is a stage beyond desires when one has a true understanding of one's true self (*Atmabodha*).

The experience of hypnosis and *dhyana* originate in 4th state of consciousness, called *Turya* or the transcendental state (mentioned as Supermind by Rohit Mehta (1987) and Over mind by Rishi Aurobindo). *The Gita* does not describe simply because it is indescribable. Although there are phenomenological differences between hypnosis and *dhyana*. The hypnotherapist makes the subject experience the 4th state of consciousness *Turya*. When practiced as self hypnosis takes the subject further to meditation and further to the path of *Samadhi*. While in *Dhyana* or Meditation, the subject himself or herself attains the 4th state *Turya* and moves on the path forward to *Samadhi*. Both lead to ultimate liberation and self-realization. Vyas & Vyas (2021), emphasize the role of a fifth dimension or space-time consciousness continuum to explain the phenomenon of hypnosis and other paranormal occurrences.

Sri Aurobindo (1999) believed hypnosis acts on the subliminal sense of mind at the level of the inner being (Basu & Miovic, 2022). It would be not out of place to note that Patanjali's *Yoga Sutra* mentions 7 states of consciousness which is further elaborated in detail in *Yoga Vashishtha*. Hypnosis can also access all 7 aspects of the subconscious and unconscious mind clarified by Vyasa, as a commentary on *Yoga Sutra* that include individual *samskaras*, specific *samskaras* (prenatal or hereditary), unexpressed data memories stored in the collective unconscious, preprogrammed reflexes, *pranic* or bio-plasmic energy, innate fluctuations of the mind designed to change with cosmic rhythm, and finally, the psychic or supernatural powers which tend to take place in the domain of the collective unconscious.

Finally, Prof Amlan Sen was run through a hypnotherapeutic process and its relevance with respect to the Bhagavad *Gita. In the end, I discovered that although not planned there was an unplanned therapeutic process which was essentially Ericksonian.*

The Ericksonian Psychotherapeutic Process: In reference to a therapeutic context, it is essential for the hypnotherapist to understand the contextual reference of the therapy (in terms of space and time) and have an intuitive understanding of the problem of the client. *The Gita* exhorts that all subjective perceptions distort the objects of perception and knowledge involves the knower, the known, and the process of knowing. Thus, the concepts of expression (*kshetra*) and experience (*kshetragn*a) are discussed with reference to the field and the knower of the field and once these dimensions are understood, it becomes easy to commence therapy. A hypnotherapist should also have a proper understanding of the nature of the 5-fold factors of actions mentioned in *The Gita.* They are *adhisthanam* or motive, *karta* or actor, *karnam* or instruments, *chesta* or patterns of behaviour, and *daivam* or the unpredictable elements. Through *abhyasena* (practice) and *vairagya* (detachment), these need to be inculcated in therapy, and throughout the *Gita*, we witness hypnotherapy in action.

From Ego Strengthening to Ego Purification: *The Gita* stresses the need for control of the mind because the mind can both become the best friend as well as the greatest enemy (*B.G.*, *6.6*). Even if the mind is difficult to control (*B.G.*, *6.34*), the comforting news is that it can be controlled through suitable practice (*B.G.*, *6.35*). *The Gita* says that the mind is the 6th organ (***manah sasti indriyani***) and the Upanishads say that mind alone is the cause of bondage and liberation of the human being (***manahi eva manushyanama, Karanam bandh-mokshabhayoho***). One of the ways to address issues in the mind is through ego strengthening which is often used in hypnotherapy and in *The Gita* ego strengthening is used to bring Arjuna out of his depressed state. Classical hypnotherapy utilized the use of Hartland's' Ego Strengthening process. Krishna, however, is not content with mere ego boosting. He not only uses psychoanalysis, but he also uses psychosynthesis—making the mind integrated and whole leading to ego purification. Like a true therapist, Krishna helps Arjuna to first comprehend and then transcend the 3 *gunas*.

Milton Erickson was a master in the usage of Indirect communication which he found to be more effective than other forms of hypnotherapy prevalent in his times. He intentionally wanted his language pattern to be "artfully vague", abounding with the use of ambiguity because he understood that such a linguistic approach helped one in both trance induction and therapeutic application. Erickson did not pre-plan his therapy and rarely treated his patients in the same way as he believed that every patient is unique and so are their perceptive nature and solution to their problem. Most often he would use his intuitive capabilities and also rely on the principles of Observation and Utilization of the client's conscious and unconscious behaviour. This power of observation, very essential for hypnotherapists, is a measure of the level of an individual human being's ability to notice and therefore, structure a beneficial healing strategy. Therapy begins only when one is able to observe the conditioning process and once that is done, the process of deconditioning can be initiated.

A hypnotherapist primarily works on the level of the unconscious mind because he knows that as a multi-tasking system, the unconscious is trusted for its problem-solving capabilities, allowing it to work by providing only general, "**artfully vague**" commands (Valenzuela, 2015). An example of an **open-ended and vague suggestion** is when Arjuna was told by Krishna that all the men he dreaded to have been killed were already dead. This has an effect of a **double bind** which is used effectively in hypnotherapy. A bind is a question or statement that gives the client an illusion of a choice because irrespective of whatever one chooses the results are designed to be the same. In Ericksonian hypnotherapy, binds and double binds are used to lead the client in a therapeutic direction while giving one an illusion of a choice. While a bind is addressed at a conscious level, a double bind is aimed at one's unconscious. This gives the client a sense of power and freedom to choose one's way of changing and is therapeutically very effective.

Fight without any fear because I have already killed Dronacharya, Bheeshma, Jayadratha, Karna, and other brave warriors. You will win if you fight. (B.G.,11.34)

Also, in hypnotherapy, as a part of ego strengthening process, **motivational epithets** are carefully planted in suggestions. Throughout the *Gita*, one notices these motivational epithets which lend a trance-inducing characteristic. Thus, to motivate Arjuna, Krishna uses powerful adjectives, some of which are the following: *Anagha* (sinless one), *Bharatashreshta & Bharatsattama* (Best of Bharatas), *Dehabhritan Vara* (Supreme among the embodied), *Dhananjaya* (Winner of wealth), *Kirtin* (Diademed One), *Kurupravira* (Great hero of the Kurus), *Mahabaho* (mighty-armed), *Parantapa* (Scorcher of foes), *Purusharishabha* (Flower among men), *Purushavyaghra* (Tiger among men), *Sabyasachi* (One who wields the bow with either hand), etc.

In Ericksonian hypnotherapy, often the therapists suggest that the client **hold back a desired response.** When a desired response is frustrated, it increases the motivation in a client to have it all the more. Holding back, one's desired state also validates the client's present state. Arjuna wanted to see the Universal Form—the visible embodiment of the Unseen Divine. He has understood the mystery of the seen and now he wants to understand the embodiment of the Unseen Divine. But while Arjuna requests Krishna, the hypnotherapist, to demonstrate his cosmic form, Krishna does not immediately oblige. Krishna has to prepare him with the extension of sensory perception into the realms that are extra-sensory because He understood that for Arjuna to explore the Timeless Moment and to see all in One the vast expanse of Time and Space need to be explored. Krishna had to grant a special vision—a cosmic vision to experience a cosmic hypnosis.

Thou cannot behold Me with this human eye. I will bestow on thee the supernatural eye. (Divyam dadami te chakshuh). (B.G.,11.8)

Krishna while demonstrating his huge *Viswarup* form, first instils and then removes the frightful experience to address Arjun's phobia. This is a technique of **hypnotic desensitization** used by Cognitive hypnotherapists to handle phobia in patients where the therapist gradually exposes the object of fear (often on an imagined object) while experiencing relaxation. This is an effective procedure as the hypnotherapist uses relaxation, dissociation, or time distortion to counteract any possible relapse of fear.

Krishna however, soon takes Arjuna out of trance once he realizes that the goal is achieved.

***Do not be troubled; do not fear my terrible form. Let your heart be satisfied and your fears dispelled by looking at Me as I was before.* (*B.G., 11.49*)**

Here, there is also the experience of **ratification of the trance phenomena** by Arjuna in the form of catalepsy, anaesthesia, and amnesia. Arjuna was transfixed with fear in visualizing the terrible form of the Lord and had no feelings about who he was and where he was to go. As powerful convincers of a good trance experience, hypnotherapists often use strategies like amnesia, symptom substitution, hypnotic confusion, etc. They are very effective therapeutically also.

***Having seen Your many mouths bearing Your terrible teeth, resembling the raging fire at the time of annihilation, I forget where I am and do not know where to go.* (*B.G., 11.25*).**

Another technique used by hypnotherapists is forward progression and **future pacing or pre-cognition**. Effectively during hypnosis, the client gets acquainted with one of the dominant future possibilities which arise from the core of the subconscious, which obviously has immense therapeutic benefits. During *Viswarupadarshan*[18], a frightened Arjuna could visualize the future of the people for whom he was so concerned to fight. It is the *Viswarupa darshan* where Arjuna is given a preview of the Great War and what lies in the future so far as the Kurukshetra war is concerned.

***I see all the sons of Dhritarashtra and their supporting kings, with Bhisma, Drona, and Karna and also our soldiers, hurtling helplessly into Your sinister mouth. Your terrible teeth crushing their heads. I see our warriors and all the kings who are here to fight. All are rushing into your awful jaws; I see them crushed by your teeth.* (*B.G., 11.26-27*)**

The **use of repetitions**—stories, concepts, and words—is widely used as a technology in hypnosis—used both to reinforce depth in trance and generate positive therapeutic outcomes. In the *Gita*, Krishna uses the same idea repeatedly in all the chapters to reinforce a therapeutic effect. The second chapter of the *Gita*, *Samkhya Yoga*, is in a sense the essence and summary of the entire *Gita* which contains ideas repeated throughout the *Gita's* remaining chapters. The use of repetition (*punarukti*) is skilfully used by the therapist to transplant an idea into the unconscious skilfully and without the client's conscious awareness. The concept of the soul is repeated in many places in the *Gita*. For the *guru* in Krishna, repetitions are often done to ensure that the spiritual principles are grasped deeply.

Also, the topic of transcending the three kinds of *gunas* (*sattvic, rajasic, and tamasic*) is explained in Chapter 17 and also again in Chapter 18 of the *Gita*. Likewise, the idea of surrender is repeated.

Always think of Me, be devoted to Me, worship Me, and offer obeisance to Me. Showing such devotion, you will surely reach Me. (B.G., 9.34)

Focus your mind on Me. Become my devotee. Worship Me. Offer your obeisance to Me. Then certainly you will attain Me. It's my promise to you because you are very dear to me. (B.G., 18.65).

It is worthwhile to note that while there are similarities in both sentences, in the later verse Krishna stresses the context and content. He explains specifically what the seeker needs to do to attain Him. Krishna also mentions what He was going to offer as a guarantee because his devotees are very dear to Him (*priyo si me*). This feature is called **Reframing Technique** in hypnotherapy, which is a technique of changing mental frames, ideas, and beliefs and is effectively used by Ericksonian hypnotherapists.

Like repetition, another effective technique used by hypnotherapists is the **principle of distraction and pattern intervention**. These have a trance-inducing effect and has also great therapeutic significance. In the first chapter, when Arjuna was overwhelmed with grief, guilt, fear, and hopelessness, Krishna had to apply the principle of distraction and pattern intervention to therapeutically address the objective by directing Arjuna to the rightful action which was done by deliberating switching topics and changing Arjuna's focus and attention.

An Ericksonian hypnotherapist uses metaphors extensively creating stories that somehow match the client's experience. Thus, metaphors must be isomorphic in the sense that somehow, they should resemble the client's situation, problem, experience, goal, etc. (Gordon,1978). Also, analogies are used extensively to tell stories about other people who have had similar problems or issues. One such technique is the 'My friend Jack' technique used effectively by Ericksonian hypnotherapists when they use analogies of the therapist's friends to subconsciously drive a point.

Symbols are similar to metaphors in that they represent something else. They are, however, concrete objects or representations, standing for abstract ideas or concepts. The example of **symbolism** in the *Gita* starts from the very first line and the first two words itself. The first two words—*Dharmashetra Kurukshetra*—start symbolically representing the conflict at various levels which is to follow in the entire *Gita*. They refer to religious and spiritual duties and activities as contrasted with mundane responsibilities and activities. It starts with duality—*Kurukshetra* is represented by Dhritarashtra and his narrow mentality against *Dharmashetra* of the Pandavas and Krishna Himself.

It would be interesting to note that most of the names in the *Gita* represent either a psychological tendency or metaphysical principles, designed to subtly touch the unconscious. Some of the examples are: *Dhritarasthra* is one who upholds the kingdom (of the senses); *Sanjaya* represents one who is completely victorious; *Duryodhana* is one who is hard to be countered in any way or one who uses unscrupulous means to get what he wants and *Drona* implies that which remains melted—a powerful force of habitual tendencies.

Some examples of the use of metaphors, similes, and symbols are outlined below:

Like a tortoise pulls his limbs into his shell, one keeps his senses under one's control. **(*B.G.*, *2.58*)**

***Just as the rivers entering the ocean cannot disturb the ocean in any way, desires to enter the mind cannot disturb the steady mind of a sage.* (*B.G., 2.70*)**

***Excessive desire can cover the mind's clarity just as smoke covers fire, dust covers a mirror, and the womb covers a foetus.* (*B.G., 3.38*)**

A sensitive mind is like a mirror—it reflects but gathers dust. Here, it is to be noted that the usage of a mirror represents consciousness, and only an individual who is clean like a mirror can be unattached and aware of it. Mirror exercises are also used by hypnotherapists in visualization trances to therapeutically unravel different dimensions of one's personality and experience dissociation at multiple levels. This dissociative effect helps one to objectively view the context of one's problem along with the myriad solution possibilities.

The *Gita* is replete with the usage of symbols in all 18 chapters. They can be very effective if they are included as part of subtle and embedded suggestions. Some examples are:

***Just as we discard old, worn-out clothes, the soul casts off worn-out bodies to enter a new body at the time of death. A body is for the soul what clothes are for us.* (*B.G., 2.22*)**

***Just as a big lake can minimize the importance of a small well, so does the knower of the absolute truth proficient in Shastras serve better than the Vedas.* (*B.G., 2.46*)**

***When ignorance is destroyed by true knowledge, God is revealed. Just as the sun heralds visibility in the daytime.* (B.G., 5.16)**

***As the air carries fragrance from place to place, so does the soul carry its mind and perceptions from body to body.* (*B.G., 15.8*)**

***No one should abandon duties because he sees defects in them. Every action, every activity, is surrounded by defects as a fire is surrounded by smoke.* (*B.G., 18.48*)**

In chapter 15, the first few verses refer to the symbol of an inverted banyan tree which has its roots growing upwards and branch downwards. Nurtured by the three *gunas*, the branches spread downwards and upwards. The roots are bound by *karma*, the fruitive activities of human beings.

In the *Gita*, Arjuna in the last chapter wakes up from a deep trance-like state. He gets his memory back (*smriti labdha*). It would be interesting to note that during a session, the Ericksonian hypnotherapist often uses an **amnesia gap** by using the same word or phrase before and after a suggestion. To keep a client from blocking, disturbing, or even destroying unconscious changes, Ericksonian hypnotherapists often create amnesia for the trance experience, unlike traditional hypnotherapists. Thus, the imagery of the hair is skilfully used to create amnesia for the therapy. While it was used at the beginning of the first chapter (*roma-harshash cha jayate*) during trance induction, it was also used again in the last chapter at the time of trance termination (*roma-harshanam*) thereby creating amnesia of the therapeutic context in between. The changes that occurred within Arjuna during the period of the entire 18 chapters (single session therapy) operated at a deeper unconscious level.

In terms of meeting the psychotherapeutic outcome in the *Gita*, the last chapter is a manual for cognitive hypnotherapists whose primary vocation is to trigger possible solution options from the client without being directive and specific. Lord Krishna played the role of a catalyst in clearing all forms of doubts in Arjuna's mind and once all doubts were cleared, Arjuna decided to pick up the bow and fight. Krishna merely concurred with his decision. This was the insightful and intuitive spark of wisdom in Arjuna—the ability to have a perception of the whole that transcends knowledge which is the seeing of the parts.

***Thus, the Wisdom which is a greater secret than all secrets has been declared to you by Me; having reflected upon it fully you now act as you choose.* (*B.G., 18.63*)**

Krishna was indicating to Arjuna his *swadharma*[19], which he was resisting because he was not able to see his own *swabhava.*[20] Once the perception of his true nature came to him, he spontaneously chose the path that was indicated to him and this is the intuitive realization that happens in hypnosis.

First, Krishna not only articulates the goal of therapy but like a perfect therapist, explains the consequences of a wrong decision.

***If you still refuse to fight this dharmic battle, you are sinning by not performing your duty. You will lose your reputation too.* (*B.G., 2.33*)**

Sometimes, the hypnotherapist needs to cross-validate the therapeutic outcome from the client.

***O Partha, have you been hearing my words with concentration? Are your ignorance and illusion destroyed as yet, O' Dhananjaya?* (*B.G., 18.72*)**

And eventually, it is followed by a grateful response from the client.

***My delusion is gone! I have regained memory of my soul through Thy grace, O Achyuta.*[21] *I am firmly established; my dubiousness has vanished. I will act accordingly to thy word.* (*B.G., 18.73*)**

The *Gita* closes with a universal, transcendental message for all mankind and all ages.

***Wherever there is Krishna, the master of all mystics, and wherever there is Arjuna, the supreme archer, there will also certainly be opulence, victory, extraordinary power, and morality. That is my opinion.* (*B.G., 18.78*).**

This assertion is a form of post-hypnotic suggestion used in hypnotherapy, which is a condition in which one who has been previously deeply hypnotized, will accept suggestions similar to hypnotic ones, without having been subjected to any further hypnotic process or having passed through any state resembling sleep or trance. This is the impact on us and anyone (like Arjuna, Sanjaya, Dhritarashtra, and others) who has cherished the profound message of the *Gita*.

This was earlier reflected in the most oft-quoted *shloka*:

***Whenever and wherever there is a decline in religious practice, O descendant of Bharata, and a predominant rise of irreligion—at that time I descend Myself.* (*B.G., 4.7*)**

Conclusion

Hypnotherapy is gradually generating interest among psychotherapy practitioners and there is a positive movement towards intervention which values innate human and subjective experiences. Compassionate Ericksonian hypnotherapy popularized by Stephen Brooks has been able to garner a lot of interest throughout the globe because it has been successfully able to marry Western psychotherapy with Eastern mysticism. Psychology and psychotherapy cannot be effective without the spiritual and "psyche" (In Greek meaning soul) component. Also, there is a lot of positive interest generated in areas like Psychoneuroimmunology and the psychobiology of beliefs along with Consciousness-based studies in healing and therapy. Indian universities and Medical colleges should include Indian Hypnotherapy in course curricula for medical practitioners, psychologists, and psychotherapists so that future generations can reap the benefits of the art and science of this wonderful domain. While trying to appreciate the use of the metaphors in The *Gita*, one cannot but overlook that The *Gita* has also been used as a metaphor for psychotherapeutic healing and spiritual transcendence.

Notes

1. *Sanatana* tradition.
2. Equanimity.
3. Purification of the mind.
4. Bereavement.
5. *Vedantic* doctrine of non-duality.
6. Discernment or discrimination.
7. Equal or even.
8. Discipline at the verbal level.
9. Self-realization.
10. Liberation.
11. A work of sacred scripture in Hinduism.
12. Alternative name for Hinduism. Literally means eternal religion.
13. Relating to or of *dharma.*

14. Faith.
15. Student.
16. Hindu religious training or discipline through which an individual attains *samadhi*.
17. Self-learning.
18. Witnessing Lord Krishna's universal form.
19. Practicing own *dharma*.
20. Intrinsic nature of an individual.
21. One who will never lose his inherent nature and powers.

References

Aurobindo (1999). *Synthesis of Yoga.* Shri Aurobindo Trust: Pondicherry, India.

Avasthi, A., Kate, N. & Grover, S. (2013). "Indianization of Psychiatry Utilizing Indian Mental Concepts", *Indian Journal of Psychiatry*, 55 (S136-144). DOI: 10.4103/0019-5545.105508

Bhawuk, D.P.S, (2011). *Spirituality and Indian Psychology: Lessons from the Bhagavad-Gita.* Springer: London.

Dey, A.C. (1955). *Message of Godhead.* https://www.prabhupada-media.net/book-pdf/1955-Message_of_Godhead.pdf

Durant, W. & Durant, A. (1937). *The Story of Civilization,* p. 931. Impact Global Publishing.

Easwaran, E. (1997). *The Gita for Daily Living.* Jaico Publishing House: New Delhi.

Gordon, D. (1978). *Therapeutic Metaphors.* Meta Publications.

Malhotra, R. & Babaji, S. D. (2020). *Sanskrit Non-translatable: The Importance of Sanskritizing English.* Manjul Publishing House: New Delhi.

Max Muller, F. & Bloomfield, M. (1897). *The Interpretation of History.* Gyan Publishing House: India.

Mehta, R. (1987). *The Secret of Self-transformation: A Synthesis of Tantra and Yoga.* Motilal Banarsidass Publishers: New Delhi.

Mehta, R. (1995). *From Mind to Super-mind: A Commentary on the Bhagavad Gita.* Motilal Banarisadass Publisher: New Delhi.

Panda, N.C. (2003). *Yoga-Nidra: Yogic trance, Theory, Practice, and Applications.* Delhi, India: DK Printworld.

Patra, D. & Neelakandan, R. (2021). "Yoga Nidra and Hypnotherapy: Powerful Healing Modalities for the Future". *UIJIR,* Vol. 2 (4). DOI No.—08.2020-25662434.

Prabhupada, B.S. (1999). *The Path of Yoga.* Bhaktivedanta Book Trust: Kolkata.

Rao, V. (1980). "*Gita* & Mental Sciences". *Indian Journal of Psychiatry, 22*: 19-31.

Reddy, M.S. (2012). "Psychotherapy—Insights from the Bhagavad Gita". *Indian Journal of Psychological Medicine, 34*(1).

Saraswati, S.S. (1976). *Yoga Nidra.* Yoga Publications Trust: Munger.

Valenzuela, F.O. (2015). *Psycho-Oncology, Hypnosis and Psychosomatic Healing in Cancer*. Trafford Publishing: USA.

Vivekananda, S. (1947). *Complete Works of Swami Vivekananda.* Advaita Ashram: Kolkata.

Vyas, B. & Vyas, R. (2009). *Indian Handbook of Hypnotherapy: Foundations and Strategy.* Concept Publishing Company: New Delhi.

Vyas, B. & Vyas, R. (2017). *Contemporizing Raj Yoga: Neuroscience and Practices.* Concept Publishing Company: New Delhi.

Vyas, B. & Vyas, R. (2021). *Space-time Consciousness: Rationale of the Paranormal.* Concept Publishing Co, Pvt. Ltd.: New Delhi.

Yogananda (2002). *The Gita: God talks with Arjun: The Royal Science of God Realization*. Yogoda Satsanga Society of India: Kolkata.

5

Hypnotherapeutic Processes and Techniques

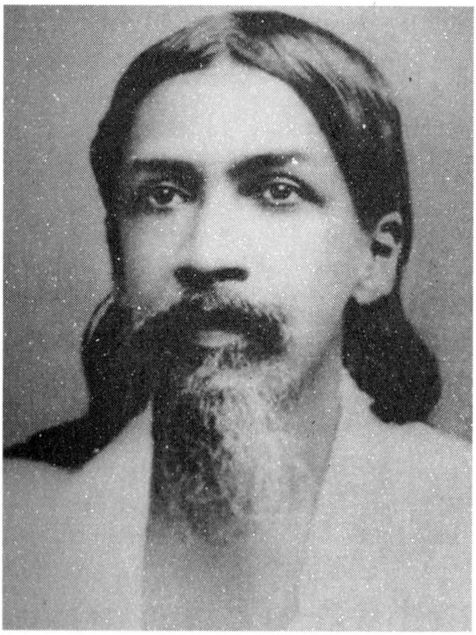

A DREAM OF SURREAL SCIENCE
By Sri Aurobindo Ghosh
Collected Poems of Sri Aurobindo

One dreamed and saw a gland write Hamlet; drink
At the Mermaid, capture immortality;
A committee of hormones on the Aegean's brisk
composed Iliad and the Odyssey.

A thyroid, meditating almost nude under the Iliad tree,
Saw the eternal light,
And arising from its mighty solitude,
Spoke of the wheel and eightfold path alright.

A brain by a disordered stomach driven
Thundered through Europe, conquered, ruled and fell,
From St. Helena, went perhaps to Heaven.

Thus wagged on the surreal world, until
A scientist played with atoms and blew out
The Universe before God had time to shout.

Innovation would be the mother of invention. Every therapist is recommended to tailor the strategy for an individual client/ patient as per the attitude and problems of the patient. However, it is appreciated that a novice would find this difficult. Even command hypnotherapy also works. Therefore, where we have succeeded in producing successful results during the course of 40+ years of our hypnotherapeutic practice, we reproduce the sessions verbatim. What was said as a conclusion in previous chapters is repeated here. Milton Erickson has done so much for hypnotherapy. His success is still available to the novice so as to use river, sea, mountains, hills, trees, forests, and the leaves, etc. as archetypal symbols. What Freud elucidated in his masterpiece as 'Interpretation of Dreams' in 1899 is still relevant to entire mankind and maybe utilized as symbols in trance. Yet, the 21st century demands a further contemporization that is the relevance of this book.

Meditative practice with an alternative title as *Raj Yoga* has found universal acceptance. Meditative practice is said to be spiritual but it is not entirely a domain for the spiritual. That also generates better health and a spiritual person will be more spiritual.

The meditator experiences a different state that ancient scriptures call *'Turya'*.

Hypnotherapy is also getting better and better acceptance in India. The widespread misbelief that it was some kind of evil practice to hoodwink people has disappeared. The hypnotherapists have found themselves as a special kind of therapist that may or may not use minimal drugs. For hypnosis there are 3 levels that are well charted: Light, medium and deep. For research, further levels of the state of trance range up to 12 both in Harvard and Stanford hypnotic susceptibility test. But, for a hypnotherapist in clinical mode, even a light trance does produce results.

Axioms

There is still a lot to understand about consciousness. Therefore, hypnosis that is an altered state of consciousness has yet to be philosophically deciphered. As we have seen earlier that even a profound sage Maharshi Aurobindo had opinions. The relevance of any opinion for a scientific mode has to be validated in a laboratory with varying scientists and different locations. We just want a hypnotherapist to excel and the excellence when he is able to cure/ benefit a wide spectrum of his patients.

We avoid further philosophical reflections. Instead we derive certain axioms that should be taken as granted. A therapeutic strategy respecting the axioms is most likely to produce a successful result for the patient.

Hypnosis and Hypnotherapy

- Hypnosis is altered state of consciousness. It is distinctly different from other three ordinarily well known three states viz. awake, sleep and dream.
- Hypnosis is easy to induce. Anyone can learn to induce hypnosis.
- Most humans can be hypnotized. Those who resist and challenge should be avoided.

- Hypnotherapy is strategic. Such applications of hypnosis require scientific understanding of physiology and psychology. Training and practice that evolves over a number of years are a must for therapist.
- For strategic application of hypnotherapy, diagnosis of the condition being treated is necessary; so is the understanding of pathogenesis.
- Goals as well as intermediate aims in therapy need to be defined at the onset of treatment.
- Familiarity and ability to elicit various phenomena is a must for the therapist.
- The deft application of a particular phenomenon facilitates the treatment. The therapist decides which phenomenon to be invoked.
- Hypnotic state is a state characterized by heightened suggestibility. There is uncritical acceptance of the suggestion.
- The suggestions work like a surgeon's knife.
- It is the duty of the therapist to look after the physical comfort of a hypnotized subject as much as an anesthetist looks after the anesthetized patient.
- In hypnosis, there is innate preference for the natural state of well beings as well as towards positive, good and ethical aspects.
- Rapport is basic to all forms of psychotherapy. Minimum effort is necessary in hypnotherapy. Rapid and intense rapport is fundamental to the success.
- A hypnotherapist should understand that self hypnosis and meditation are similar. Let a subject take a programme suitable to his sensibilities. He may then keep on practicing this for a long, long time. He may then select the terminology to his choice.

Mind

- There is no substance to the mind; never mind, as long as we mind our mind to manipulate the mind of the subject carefully.

- There is no specific location of mind in the brain. Different centres perceive sensorial inputs at specific locations. Summation of sensorial inputs generates perception. Out of numerous and variable perceptions, concepts are generated. Mind is sixth sense organ. Concepts are basic to intelligence
- Concepts are the guidelines for function. Valid concepts provide smooth functioning at societal and personal level. Corruption of the conceptualization is basic to psychopathology. It is well said in *Upanishads* that mind alone is the cause of bondage and freedom for the human beings.
- There is no duality between mind and body. Though apparently it means that mind and body are separate entities, this is a fallacy. One is not separate from the other. There is a mind body continuum; one influences the other continuously and simultaneously.
- French philosopher Descartes was wrong in considering mind as separate from the body but his philosophy still pervades in propagating the wrong notion.
- However, Descartes was absolutely correct to say that body mechanisms function as interconnected wheels so that motion in any system sets up a dynamic movement all over.
- Unconscious mind constitutes about 90+% the psychic contents.
- Subconscious mind is the portion of psyche that can be brought into awareness with some effort, constitutes about 4 to 6%
- Conscious mind, that is ordinary aware, constitutes about 3 to 4% of psyche.

Physiology and Pathogenesis

- Homeostasis, i.e. a continuous maintenance of equilibrium of all the parameters at molecular and systemic levels is fundamental to life.

- An aberration in any of the parameters causes a disorder or a disease.
- An infection in the body produces a particular disease. A perpetual conceptual corruption causes psychic disturbance so as to produce stress. This is basic to psychosomatic diseases.
- Psychic disturbances can be behavioural, cognitive or both.
- Corrupt conceptualization is like a virus. It can crash all the data.
- Psychological disorders and organic diseases are understood at molecular level; however these levels by themselves do not constitute a disorder or a disease. Mere biochemical correction does not reverse the disease process.
- Psychodynamic discreativity either creates the disease or contributes to its propagation. Most disorders/diseases arise from the faulty functioning of discriminative wisdom. This quote from Charaka summarizes the etiopathology of most disorders/diseases.
- Diseases are the metaphors that body creates to express its discomfort because of a traumatized mind.
- Thoughts and emotions equate with floating particles in blood stream.
- Emotions are further identified with numerous biochemical substances such as hormones, neurotransmitters and other information substances.
- Symptoms arise when events are inadequately processed so that there is repression into unconscious mind.
- Unconscious mind is the hidden dynamo that drives the bodily functions most of the times.

Therapeutic Process

- Belief is fundamental to therapeutic cure. One who doubts, perishes was said in *Bhagavad Gita*.
- Hypnotherapy is the therapy of new millennium.
- Hypnotherapy is drugless therapy: Progress has begun

with the movement in New Age, however drugs do have a justified use and should not be excluded.

- Hypnotherapist cannot lie. However, he puts bitter truths in sugarcoated form. You will speak the truth; but speak it in pleasant, acceptable way.
- The therapist should be focalized during the session.
- Expectancy, novelty and wonders and continuous building up of them is one of the most important ingredients in therapy.
- Therapy aims at relief or cure: there is no judgment of the patient/client.
- Values of the client, personal or cultural are his/her property. They have to be respected and so honoured. Use the currency of the country you are in during the proceedings.
- During hypnosis, an event may be relived; so that the memory can be erased or modified. Reliving a happy event can provide substitution for the traumatic one.

Dynamics of Change

- Suggestions work, since in hypnosis, surreal is identified as real. This is reinforced by the therapist. Metaphors are surreal symbols.
- Language, semantically as well as through syntax, is understood by brain. Word is a symbol. During hypnosis, a symbol can change its meaning.
- Arousal of emotions potentiates therapy. As is the experience, so are the feelings As you feel, so it happens.
- Overall therapeutic stress reduction leads to easier maintenance of homeostasis.
- Therapeutic reversal of aberrant psychodynamics by elimination/modification of faulty perception.
- Insight generation. A moment sees what the ages toil to express.

Dynamics of Transformation: Plausible Hypotheses

- Creativity is geared to a higher order and may be, to a radically different mode.
- Neurons do not regenerate; however, brain undergoes plasticity through development of new synapses; this may be facilitated by hypnotic process.
- Changes in the conditioned/stereotype pathways in the brain.
- Opening of different functional areas of brain, such as prefrontal cortex and downgrading of function of other areas. fMRI studies will prove.
- Melatonin level will prove.
- Different gene expression studies can prove.

Original Sanskrit sentences are removed from the main text. They can be found below if interested:

- *Pragyna aparadha jayate sarve rogan* (All diseases arise from the faulty functioning of discriminative wisdom. This quote from Charaka summarizes the etiopathology of all diseases).
- *Sanshayatma Vinashyati.* One who doubts perishes.
- *Satyam bruyat, priyam bruyat* (You will speak the truth; but speak it in pleasant, acceptable way).
- *Yad bhava, tad bhavana; yad bhavana, tad bhavatu.* As is the experience, so are the feelings As you feel, so it happens.
- *Manah shasti indriyani.* Mind is sixth sense organ.
- *Manah eva manushyanam karanan bandh mokshabhyoho.* Mind alone is the cause of bondage and freedom for the human beings.

Innovations in technique

Induction Techniques

There are numerous techniques available for induction. Besides being lengthy, some of them are lackluster. Novelty, wonder and some luminosity facilitates induction to go faster. We therefore mention only those who have above qualities in addition to time saving.

1. **Induction by PMR and deep breathing (simple technique)**. Progressive muscular relaxation is being taught as a standard method for trance induction. However, the method is time consuming. We have therefore advocated the following time saving induction methods:
2. **Induction by pendulum**
3. **Induction by coin technique**
4. **Induction by electromagnetic two hands technique as formulated by Ernest Rossi**

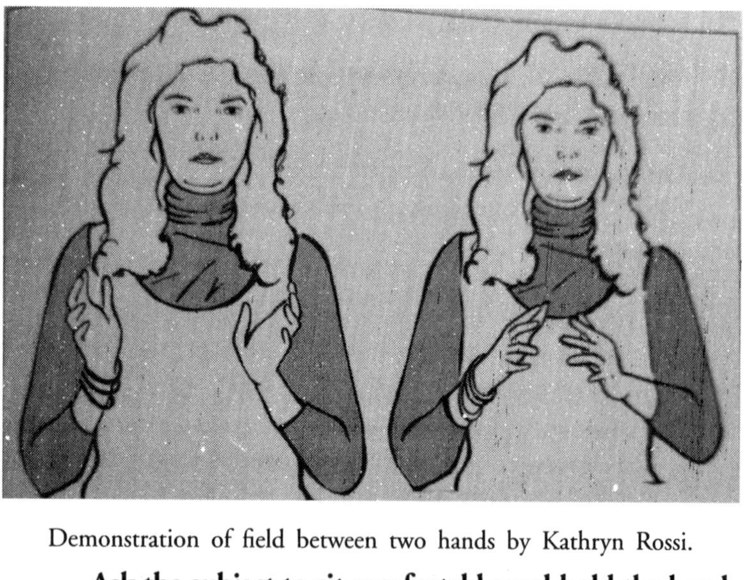

Demonstration of field between two hands by Kathryn Rossi.

Ask the subject to sit comfortably and hold the hands straight at the shoulder level about 14 inches apart. Ask them to oscillate the hands a few inches towards each other and as he does that, perceive that with every move towards each other, it is gradually getting difficult to draw them apart. They move closer and closer with each oscillation so that they come to clasp each other

eventually. It is difficult to separate them now. Apply some force to unclasp them and still they remain stuck. Suggest that as the therapist separates them, they do so easily and fall in the lap. Trance ensues.

Quick induction technique by athetoid movement of one hand; confusion technique—The subject is just asked to relax. No explanation is provided when athetoid movement at any of the hands at shoulder, elbow, wrist and some fingers are executed passively. The patient is left wondering what is happening. The state of wonder is highly conducive to induction of trance.

5. **For children—favourite cartoon may be used and a story that grandma would have used may also be helpful**

To confirm whether the subject is in trance (light, moderate or deep) is to be assessed for suggestions of the condition.

Confirmation of light trance

1. When subject tries to open the eyes
2. Fluttering of eyes
3. Not comfortable in any position
4. Showing anxiety for closing eyes

Confirmation of moderate trance is by:

1. Ideomotor signalling
2. Demeanour of the subject (body language)
3. Hand levitation
4. Pulse (lower)

Deepening Technique—

1. Ask the subject to take deep breathe in and out, may be once or three four times till subject is in deep trance.
2. Asking the subject to swallow (due to sympathetic over-activation there will be dryness of lips, tongue and throat)

e.g. as you will swallow, you will feel comfortable, quiet and tranquil within yourself.

3. Make yourself more comfortable by moving your shoulder or any other part of your body where you are feeling discomfort.
4. The subject is asked to open the eyelids. When he is finding it difficult, reinforce that difficulty is a good symptom that the trance progresses better when the eyelids cannot open at all.

Confirmation of Deep trance

1. Experience a virtual reality, e.g.
   - Fragrance of perfume.
   - Felt descending steps.
   - Felt warm breeze on cheek.
2. Experience time dilation, usually shortened.
3. Eyelids cannot be opened.
4. Hand goes up in air; it can remain up for longer duration.
5. Hypno anaesthesia.

Depending on severity of the condition that one is trying to treat, you may need to deepen often during the session.

When the subject is treated for any symptoms, he/she works at unconscious level. When the work is going on, reliving occurs. All the memory starts replaying. The subject starts re-experiencing it. He/she becomes lighter in trance and starts waking up. So deepening becomes necessary. Various situation occurs like trying to open the eyes, moving the fingers or any part of the body, trying to get alert, or even catharsis such as sobbing, crying, rolling on the ground, or certain violent behaviours, etc.

Depending upon the condition treated, the subject may remain in trance for a longer time. The subject is working into their unconscious. We have seen the subject remain in trance for 3 days when she was looked after by an attendant for daily routine. When she fully woke up, she said that now she has made the decision for the future. She was living in a *ashram* for more than an year. But she returned to her parents subsequently. The other phenomenon that we observed was that the subject shies away from the therapist in such a case, the suggestions for ego strengthening are given. Subject is assured to be normal functioning and follow up with this subject is done.

Conditions treated or alleviated with Hypnotherapy

Keeping in mind the safety of subjects with adequate family support, explaining the risk of leaving alone the subject, with full written consent of relation or accompanying person, we can take the treatment for the subject, to alleviate the symptoms for incurable diseases. If the subject is on traditional or alternative treatment modalities, he/she should continue the treatment and supplement it with hypnotherapy. Later on gradually, the other treatments can be withdrawn. The subject is advised to always keep their medicines.

Treatment in 1970s by Simonton and Simonton for terminally ill cancer patients waiting to die in airforce hospital is a proof that it treats and makes life comfortable or cures declared terminally sick people also. This ushered a new era for hope for cancer patients. However, this is a kind of omnibus statement; different cancers do behave differently.

Benefit for various types of pain is supported. A 1995 consensus statement by the U.S. National Institute of Health notes that, "Evidence supporting the effectiveness of hypnosis in alleviating chronic pain associated with cancer seems strong."

Indications

A. Psychological disorders

1. Stress
2. Anxiety
3. Memory Enhancement and Better study
4. Crcativity
5. Substance Abuse—Tobacco/Alcohol/Drugs, etc.
6. Insomnia
7. OCD—Obsessive Compulsive Disorder

8. Phobia
9. Mania
10. Tics
11. ADHD—Attention Deficit Hyperactivity Disorder
12. Panic attacks
13. Dissociative disorders and conversion symptom
14. Habits.

B. Psychosomatic disease/disorder

1. Migraine
2. Vertigo
3. Irritable Bowel Syndrome
4. Acidity
5. Regur*Gita*tion
6. Aerophagia
7. Trichophagia—eating of hair.
   During the residency, when hypnotherapy was not even thought of in India, we have treated and published a paper on trichobeozar. The condition recurred because we had not understood the psychodynamics.

C. Mental Illness

1. Neurosis
2. Psychosis
3. Schizophrenia—To be handled by only experts
4. Dissociative Personality Disorder
5. Possession
6. Depression.

D. Diseases of fascia/ligaments/fibrous tissue/synovial membrane

1. Cervical Spondylitis
2. Carpal Tunnel Syndrome and mesenchymal tissue disease
3. Trigger finger
4. Duputryn's contracture
5. Rheumatoid arthritis
6. Osteoarthritis
7. Temporo-mandibular joint arthritis

8. Prolapsed intervertebral disc
9. Calcaneal Spur
10. Restless Leg Syndrome: Severe night cramps in the muscles of sole/calf
11. Fibromyalgia
12. Tennis Elbow
13. Frozen Shoulder
14. Myofascial Pain Syndrome.

E. Skin disorder

1. Skin rash
2. Hyperhidrosis
3. Non-healing wound/ulcer
4. Psoriasis
5. Pemphigus
6. Alopecia
7. Blushing
8. Eczema
9. Prurities
10. Warts.

F. Gynaecological Problems

1. Menopause
2. Unexplained reproductive failure
3. PCOD
4. Dysmenorrhoea
5. Menstrual irregularities.

G. Sexual Disorders

1. Frigidity and Dysparunia
2. Hypersexuality
3. Erectile Dysfunction
4. Impotence.

H. Problems relating to relationships

1. Intermarital issues
2. Interpersonal issues.

I. Paediatric problems

1. Anxiety in Infancy
2. Child abuse and Neglect

3. ADHD (Hyperactive children)
4. Conduct Disorders
5. Separation Anxiety
6. Overanxious Disorder
7. Childhood Depression
8. Enuresis
9. Learning disabilities
10. Memory and creativity enhancement.

J. Pain Management

1. Pain—Muscular, Somatic
2. Type of Pain—Throbbing Pain, Inflammation, etc.
3. Spasmodic pain, stone or colic of abdomen
4. Trauma
5. Musculo-facial
6. Obstetric pain—Even applicable to conduct a painless delivery.
7. Cancer Pain (for symptomatic relief only).

K. Syndrome/Disorder of nerves (The swelling of the nerves is due to the edema of the sheath of the nerve bundles)

1. Trigeminal Neuralgia
2. Facial Paresis/palsy
3. Brachial Plexus Syndrome/Cervical Rib Syndrome
4. Sciatica
5. Spinal nerve compression due to prolapsed intervertebral disc.

L. Autonomic Nervous System

1. Asthma
2. Irritable Bowel Syndrome
3. Coronary heart disease.

M. Autoimmune Disorders

1. ALS—Amyotrophic Lateral Sclerosis
2. Ulcerative colitis
3. Rheumatoid Arthritis
4. Motor Neuron Disease
5. Systemic Lupus Erythematosus

6. Scelroderma
7. Polymyositis
8. Dermatomyositis
9. Sjogrens Disease and Syndrome
10. Mixed Connective Tissue disease
11. Small vessel vasculitis.

N. Misc.

1. Obesity.

O. Auto immune diseases of tissues of mesenchymal origin elsewhere

1. Dermatitis of various non-infective types, psoriasis
2. Iridocyclitis
3. Acute and chronic glomerulomyelitis.

Parkinson's disease as well as Alzheimer's disease.—The brain cells are being replaced by glial tissue in this condition. The mechanism of cell death seems to be anoxia. Whether it is glial proliferation that "strangulates and/or suffocates" the brain cells or it is secondary to the replacement of dead cells is difficult to say.

We have chiselled out a finely tuned strategy for hypnotherapy that is based on what is discussed so far as contemporizing hypnotherapy. The strategy now being used relies heavily on suggestions based on archetypal symbols relevant to the Indian ethos. This has widened the ambit of our hypnotherapeutic field, so that apart from "anecdotal success here and there", we have been having successful outcomes in a variety of conditions that range from what has been classically described to several other clinical conditions; say, success has been consistent with migraine, asthma, myofascial syndrome, irritable bowel syndrome, phobia, etc. What is noteworthy is the successful outcome in cervical rib syndrome, trigeminal neuralgia, prolapsed intervertebral disc, osteoarthritis of knees, infertility of unknown origin and such other conditions that are enumerated above.

We draw an exhaustive list of conditions, compiled by U.S. National Institute of Health where hypnotherapy has been tried with variable results. That list is truly exhaustive since it lists several hundred conditions.

The list can go on but in short understanding the etiopathology of the disease can help the subject. We can take the subject for hypnotherapy with full understanding between therapist, relations and patients.

Therapeutic Strategy

For most conditions like habit modification, symptom amelioration and psychological disorder, simple imageries usually suffice.

The imagery deployed may be:

- Symptom substitution
- Symptom transformation
- Assertiveness
- Positive imagery such as:
  Red balloon rising upwards in the sky, getting bigger, and bigger till it bursts
  Black board; scribbled, wiped clean and written and drawn stylish now
  Helmet image; for protection
  Comfort chamber; for most stressful conditions
  Ice cube melting; melting of anger
  Ice cube application; for cooling down; hypnoanaesthesia
  Sunrise; sea shore, mountains or landscape; for most stressful conditions, according to the sensibilities of the subject
  Flowers in a garden, buds opening out, all colours, VIBGYOR (violet, indigo, blue, green, yellow, orange, red)
  Germination of a seed; creativity, insight generation
  Flowing river; psychodynamics that rise, swell and normalize; flow of hormones
- Incorporation of archetypal symbols (depending upon patient's life experiences, interest and values)

Further elaboration in the strategy can be obtained by:

- Time distortion
- Age regression and cognitive restructuring
- Age progression and mental rehearsal
- Response substitution

The sessions become more complex and less structured as we proceed further to disorders of autonomic nervous system, imbalances and stress management. Hormonal disturbances and auto immune disease may need many sessions over a period of protracted therapy. The goals will also vary.

• **Theatre strategy utilizes age regression covertly.**

The subject is made to sit in a vast, comfortable, air conditioned theatre, with a remote control in his/her hand. The movie begins and the screen displays the subject and therapist to begin with.

The subject leisurely moves the remote control and movements of the clicking are utilized as ideomotor signals. It proceeds to fast backwards mode till the phobic object/situation/panic attack appears on the screen. The subject is given a solid stick by the therapist, rushes to the screen and smashes the object/situation. While the subject of the phobia is smashed, the screen is left intact. Walking back to a comfortable seat, the subject commands fast forward mode to come back, on to the screen, on the day of therapy; completely well; totally rid of phobia/panic attack. This is performed as a virtual drama during hypnotic trance.

Suggestions

The number of sessions will depend on the diagnosis, maybe with insight generation it may be 1 or long standing suppressed unconscious may require up to 8 sessions. Later on, the subject may require revision of the situation. Depending on the personality, personality type, belief system, hypnotic susceptibility, receptivity to suggestions, sincerity of the subject to practice and implement for the change, etc. suggestions need to be crafted as such:

Atheist

Suggestions relating to nature like sea, mountain, flowing river, clouds/rainbows, etc. Use any panoramic landscape that you find beautiful, a happy memory or a memorable situation will do just as well. Just make sure whatever you use is pleasant imagery.

Theist

Depending on the religion and caste/sect, the gods/goddesses like Vishnu, Shankar, Durga and other goddesses, different forms of Buddha, Tirthankar or any other deity that they worship.

Use Gods like Ganapati, Shankar, Saraswati, Jesus, Allah or any other deity from one's own belief.

For Christians, confessing before a priest.

Stress relieving suggestion

1. Going to the garden.
2. Flying in the clouds and in form of rains: de-stressing.
3. Going to the temple, flowing stream and feeding ducks/fish.
4. Cleaning up the Room or Mirror of the mind.
5. Age regression and moving the tape fast forward and backward.
6. Age progression to a state of well being and visualizing the situation/position of the person after a few years.
7. Walking through a dark jungle.
8. Mind—Computer. Comparing Hypnotherapy with PC software.
9. Cleaning of blackboard with duster.
10. Any other suggestion based on the history and personality of the subject.

Suggestions for yourself

Negative inputs like:

1. I am useless

2. Nobody likes me
3. I am a burden
4. I am a problem to all, etc.

Should be switched with positive inputs like:

1. I am OK
2. I am useful
3. I am peaceful
4. I am blissful
5. I am pure and lovable
6. I am happy, powerful and capable.

Suggestions related to the following can be utilized depending on the history and symptoms of the subject:

- **Autonomic Nervous System**
- **Hormonal Axis**
- **Happy Chemicals**
- **Biochemicals**
- **Immune System**
- **Information Substances and its action**
- **Genetic manipulation.**

Using various Metaphors, Similes, Telling stories from *Panchtantra*, *Puranas*, *Bhagavad*, poetry, Anderson tales, Hansel and Gretel, etc.

Remembering, repetition, reinforce, re-validation, re-education, re-emphasis, rejuvenation, re-learn, to get the relief by reliving and relishing the joyful memory. The self is relocated, by the relaxation everyday maybe with the help of resource person. It is a good, easy and effective remedy and health is restored.

Outline for Therapeutic Session

History taking: It is done in such a way that it builds rapport with the subject and shifts the paradigm, strengthens their ego, assesses personality profile which helps in formulating suggestions.

Name, age, education, profession, belief system of the subject are noted.

First Session

- Address the person by his/her name and make him/her comfortable, and ask him that if you have any question feel free to ask. The most important thing is that you should be comfortable and relaxed.
- This is so simple so you can take a deep and deeper breath and show me. As you take deep breath feel relax, feel more and more relax all over your body.
- And now you are taking a further deep breath, how nice and what a quick learner you are.
- Yes you are really a highly talented person to learn so quickly, learn so far.
- Yes this is a very memorable day that you have started experiencing a most wonderful state that a human being is capable of, and now take a deep breath and further deep breath.
- As you listen to my voice your eyes are getting heavier and as you take deep breath your eyes are getting heavier. Feel a wonderful state of peace, ease, calm, and cool.
- When you are experiencing the state of ease show me by moving your index finger of right hand, but if you are not experiencing any ease feel free to let me know by moving the index finger of your left hand, it's your choice.
- When there is a peace of mind, in your natural state relax even more and more. It shall be my endeavour and duty to at least make you feel comfortable, ease and peace with yourself.
- You have learned very fast and it is easy also because it is natural. You are even more relaxed than before.
- As you relax, feel comfortable, enjoy the state of wonderful alternate existence and find to feel calm, cool, and comfortable and ease.

- Because of your natural feeling so you are so touching the fundamental foundation of creativity. When I have so spoken to you, it is a great privilege for me.
- A communion in consciousness sharing that is so prevalent and I consider it to be, a great privilege that you show your confidence and you trusted me to conduct this session.
- Let's share this silence, take a deep breath in a further deeper breath state and as you feel rejuvenated any state of creative and re-creative, silence of the mind , you wake up as I count from 10 to 1.
- 10, 9, 8, 7, 6, 5, 4, 3, 2, 1, as I am counting other sounds also start back to you, listen to the sound of moving the fan, other friends are talking on the road.
- 10, 9, 8, 7, 6, 5, 4, 3, 2, 1, let me assure you that when you are coming back in your natural state of awaken.
- 9, 8, 7, 6, 5, you will feel fresh, re-fresh and cool.
- 8, 7, 6, 5, 4, to night for going to your bed, 7, 6, 5, 4, 3, before you sleep when you will lay down on the bed you will recreate this session in your mind.
- 6, 5, 4, 3, 2, you are your best friend, and when you listen to your self in this high state of creativity you experience great.
- 5, 4, 3, 2, 1, wake up and wake up awareness of your body.
- Now you totally awake as we count 5, 4, 3, 2, 1, yes very good, wonderful job, very nice, congratulations.

Termination of Trance or Waking up the subject

One has to be gentle, cool and see that he/she comes out of the trance very smoothly.

As I count from 10 to 1, 10–9–8 you will wake up. 7–6–5, the high level of your vision of high creativity and high self-esteem, it will always remain for ever. 5–4–3, S, Confidant, cheerful, creative self is you S, 3–2–1. And on arrival of 1 and you will wake up alert and wide awake.

If the subject wakes up with a complaint, treat immediately by putting the subject once again in trance and erase the symptom as it arose.

Post hypnotic Suggestions

We have utilized post hypnotic suggestions since that is a very powerful step.

- Within everyone is,
- The power to do,
- The power to know,
- The power to love,
- The difference is how one makes use of this power,
- Post hypnotic suggestions have utmost significance since they are remembered most of the time.

Methods of deepening

1. Ask the subject to take deep breath till subject settles down,
2. Repeat the last suggestion couple of times,
3. With every deep breath, you are relaxing more and more,
4. As you are listening to my voice, you are going into a deeper and deeper state of trance,
5. Your eyelids are deeply relaxed. They are very heavy. You try to open them and find that you cannot open them. ...Yes, try to open them. ...How difficult it is to open them!... And as you find you cannot open them, you go into a deeper and more peaceful state of enjoyable trance,
6. Every gesture that the subject makes, like swallowing the saliva, is utilized as: As you have swallowed that saliva, it goes down your gullet and as it goes down, you are getting down and down into a deeper state of trance,
7. Arm levitation and catalepsy of the arm,
8. Surgical anaesthesia: using glove and stocking anaesthesia induction, and
9. Insertion of a hypodermic needle.

Utilization of Deep Hypnosis for therapeutic purposes

Following hypnotic phenomena are frequently utilized as may be appropriate to the subject's symptoms:

- Time dilation and distortion, to and fro undulation of moment of time. The most frequently used method is age regression.
- Space transmigration to a comfort chamber, sea shore, mountain peaks.
- Journey through Space-time dimension.
- Goal setting by age progression.
- During trance and during post-hypnotic suggestions do not replace symptom with another symptom. Instead use the 4th state to get rid of the symptom entirely as cellular destruction happens last. First the disorder starts, then inflammation, degeneration and lastly, destruction, e.g. osteoarthritis.
- Our ancestors were aware of this process. So, beginning of stress was identified and remedial steps were taken frequently to prevent further damage.

6

Sample Scripts

Sampling a few scripts based on the techniques and strategies discussed above. Pauses and repetition are important aspects in a therapeutic session. Multiple ellipses convey a pause.

Induction Technique Sample

"I would like you to begin by just resting your back, very comfortably. You may keep your eyes open or close as you feel comfortable. Just rest your back in the way that is most comfortable for you, resting your hands on your thighs, or on the arms of the chair... . And as you just settle back... comfortably, this will be an opportunity... for you to become even more;... Yes even more; comfortable, and to experience a comfortable state. It is going to be a memorable day... memorable day... memorable day in your life.

And as you rest your back, you can begin... noticing the feelings and sensations of relaxation... a change of the feelings, and sensations of relaxation... in your body right now. Just notice some of the sensations that you can be aware of right now. For instance, you may notice the sensations in your hands as they rest there; or... perhaps you may be aware of how the chair... the chair supports your body. And as you continue listening to me... as you continue listening to me, and, breathing easily and comfortably, and deeply, de... e... ply,... take a deep... deep... deep breath in... and out... you may become aware of the sensation of comfort and relaxation as you breath, deeply, de... e... ply,... take a deep... deep... deep breath in... and out noticing that the sensations are different when you breath in... and you breathe in... and... you breathe out. Just notice those feelings as you breathe in, and fill your lungs; and... notice the sense of release of tension... , notice the sense of release of tension... as you breathe out.

How relaxed do you feel! (ID; proceed only after Yes/No response is elucidated; or repeat re-input and recapitulate the above once). To relax is to feel pleasant, at rest and at peace... would you like to feel more pleasant, more at rest and more at peace...! (ID; proceed only after Yes/No response).

And, you breathe in... and... you breathe out. Notice that a fine feeling... Notice that a fine feeling, a refined perfume... a refined perfume... of your choice... define the refined perfume of your choice... whatever it may be... you breathe in... and... you breathe out. A fine fragrance... A delicately refined fragrance... fragrance... of your choice is permeating... fragrance... of your choice is permeating... has permeated the air... in your nostrils... around your body... around your body... in the nostrils, in the lungs... all over your mind... mind... mind the smell! (ID; proceed only after Yes/No response).

Progressive Muscular Relaxation and deep breathing

And now... I want you to feel even more pleasant, more at rest and more at peace...! Would you want to feel that way? (ID; proceed only after Yes/No response).

I would like you to concentrate particularly on the relaxed feeling in sole of your feet. Just allow all the muscles and fibers in your sole and feet,... all the muscles and fibers in your feet... all the muscles and fibers in your feet... all the muscles and fibers in your soul de... e... ply relaxed.... Perhaps even picturing in your mind's eye... seeing in your mind's eye... all the muscles and fibers in your sole and feet... what they look like, for all those little muscles and tissues to relax, loosely and deeply... . R... e... l... a... x... . Allowing yourself to get that kind of feeling you have when you take off a pair of tight shoes..., .R... e... l... a... x... that you have missed for a long time... for a long time. And you can just let go of all the tension in your toes and feet, and feel the relaxation spread.

And now the... the relaxation spreads... all the muscles and fibers in your toes and feet are so re... la... xed... that... the relaxation spreads... this comfort and relaxation, is beginning to spread... spreading... and flow, like a gentle fountain of relaxation, upward spreading..., through your ankles and all through your calves... spreading... and flow, like a gentle river of relaxation... Let go all the tension in your calves, allowing them to deeply..., and, restfully..., and comfortably relax. And allow that comfort to continue, flowing upward, into your knees, and behind your knees, and through your knees, and into your thighs... spreading... and flow, like a gentle river of relaxation, letting go of all the tension in your thighs... spreading... and flow, like a gentle river of relaxation. (ID; proceed only after Yes/No response).

Perhaps, once again, imagining what that might look like, for all those large muscles and tissues, to become soft and loose, and deeply relaxed... as they bathe... in spreading... and flow, like a gentle river of relaxation... Perhaps already noticing that sense of gentle relaxation in your legs. Continue to allow that comfort to flow and spread upward, at its own pace and speed, into the front of abdomen. Flowing into your pelvis and abdomen and stomach... (Pause) through your hips and into your lower back... spreading... and flow, like a gentle river of relaxation... allow that soothing, deep comfort spread, inch by inch, up through your body, spreading from muscle group to muscle group. The abdomen is a Pandora box. There are so many organs in the abdomen. The gastrointestinal tract, the liver, spleen, the urinary tract and reproductive tract are the part of abdomen. Take a deep breathe in and out and as you take fresh energized, oxygenated energized air in, all the organs in the abdomen function properly, with great regularity and vigour.

The front and back of abdominal muscles are well relaxed. You feel very calm, cool, comfortable and tranquil in your self. Take a deep breathe in and out and relax.

Gradually, progressively flowing into your chest, into your back and into your shoulders.... Just allow all the tension to loosen, and flow away... spreading... and flow, like a gentle river of relaxation... As if somehow, every breath that you take.... And, you breathe in... and... you breathe out.... And, you breathe in... and... you breathe out... somehow, every breath you take, is just draining the end, you breathe in... and... you breathe out... taking you deeper and deeper, into comfort, with every breath you take. (ID; proceed only after Yes/No response).

And allow that comfort to flow into your neck and throat... for all little and large muscles and fibers in your neck and throat, to deeply, softly, comfortably relax... .R... e... l... a... x.... Let that relaxation go deep into your neck. And it can gradually flow up your neck, up into scalp, and all out across your scalp, as if it's just bathing your head, with waves of comfort, and relaxation... .R... e... l... a... x.... And that relaxation can flow down, into your forehead, and like a gentle wave... like a gentle river of relaxation, down across your face, into your eyes, your cheeks, your mouth and jaws like a gentle river of relaxation,.... Just let go of all the tensions in your face, your mouth, your jaws, allowing those tissues and muscles to relax..., .R... e... l... a... x.... (ID; proceed only after Yes/No response).

And now allow that comfort to flow back down your neck, and across your shoulders, and down into your arms... just relax limply and comfortably... spreading... and flow, like a gentle river of relaxation... Allow that comfort flow down from your arms, through your elbows, through your wrists, through hands, and fingers, right down through your fingertips. Let go of all the stress, and strain, all through your body. Just allowing your body to rest and relax. (ID; proceed only after Yes/No response).

The relaxation wave is now gently spreading on the Small muscles of the face. As they relax, the fresh oxygenated energised blood flows through the muscle fibers and your whole face blushes. You look 10 years younger. Just enjoy this cool fine breeze touching your cheeks... Enjoy this relaxation for a while. My voice also goes away and enjoy... . And this wave of joy and peace enters the brain, A master who controls the whole body as well as our mind and consciousness.

As the blood flows through the convolution of our brain, Energizing each and every lobe of our brain as well as all the nuclei, hormones, happy chemicals like Dopamine, Serotonin, Oxytocin etc.

You have a feeling of peace, tranquility, comfort, relax, without any stress... (ID signalling Yes/No).

Enjoy this state, a unique state of joy till you like and feeling this relaxation in your brain to stay forever. Wake up when you want and feel fresh, energized and fully relaxed."

This session is self hypnosis session to be practiced preferably in the morning and evening for 10 to 15 minutes. With practice it can be shortened to 5 minutes also.

It is also suggested that you use self hypnosis when you wake up in the morning before starting your day. It helps you get ready for a new day of various interactions (controversies) with a non-confrontational state of mind. This provides a holistic clarity in decision making and performing tasks with an equanimous mind without neurotic compensations.

Self hypnosis can be used after a day of routine interactions before sleeping so as to get rid of all the stresses of your mind before they settle into the unconscious. This helps alleviate psychosomatic conditions, like migraine, acidity, IBS, rejection or dejection of the self, etc.

The precipitation of symptoms in psychosomatic disorders is found to have many inputs. Addressing all the aspects, including the personality, the complaints, and the disease (which begins as symptoms, if not addressed multiplies) may require multiple sessions. By addressing/treating the first symptom, the unconscious ventilates and empties all other symptoms.

The subject with many symptoms should learn self hypnosis to change the personality of acceptance of what one is born of. The basic requirement of a human being is to work without expectations. (*Bhagavad Gita* 2-47. You have a right to perform your prescribed duties, but you are not entitled to the fruits of your actions). Establishing oneself in a state of 'sthitapragnya' (one with steady *pragna* or wisdom- *BG* 2 - 55-58). Reading, contemplating and understanding the second chapter of *Bhagavad Gita* helps the mind sit quietly and allow the subject to go into the 4th state of consciousness. It helps the person to be steady and without new symptoms. Subject can take the life as it is destined for himself/herself.

It has been recommended by various cultures across the world in the first phase of life, according to the choice and advice accrued by elders, teachers and family, an individual should learn and get qualified for sustenance. In the next phase, begins earning one's livelihood and should settle in life with a chosen partner. In ultimate phase of life, one will witness the fruits of their work. Settling the family and children, then one should begin withdrawing and passing on their responsibilities to the children. Finally, one should start devoting oneself to the Divine.

Self hypnosis as taught by the name *Yoga Nidra*. The scripts are as follows: (SWAMI SATYANAND MODEL)

"Welcome to *Yoga Nidra* session. Now let us warm up for *Yoga Nidra*. Please lie down on your back in *Shavasana*. (position) Cover yourself with the bed sheet. Now keep your spine and head in a straight line, with palms and the hands facing upwards and with your legs slightly apart. Adjust your body position and clothing till you are completely comfortable. Feel a sense of settling down. Please close your eyes slowly and gently. Ease yourself. Ensure that there is no stiffness or tense feeling in any part of the body. If you feel tense in any part please give a slight movement and relax.

Let us understand what *Yoga Nidra* is. It is a systematic practice for achieving total physical, mental and emotional relaxation simultaneously. It is gathering of total energy at a point in the mind. *Yoga Nidra* can be practised generally at any time of the day by any one, but in particular, after waking up in the morning and before going to bed.

Please follow the instructions without any reservations in your mind or any diversion either by way of speaking or debating with yourself. Relax your mind to become calm and quiet. Do not have any thought except for relaxation of your body and mind. There must not be any physical movement, just as you are doing before going to sleep. Please remember that this is not sleep. You are mentally alert and aware without any rigidity in the mind and body. As you closely observe your body, your mind is moving into a new realm of your consciousness. Simply listen to my words and follow.

Have a resolve in your mind with faith in the God of your choice. Repeat your resolve thrice, slowly, clearly within yourself without making any sound. Now visualise the Yoga hall from outside. Please enter the hall and visualise its ceilings, walls, windows, floor, carpet and also the space around your body. Look at your body. Your body is lying on the floor motionless. See from your head to toe and come back again from toe to head. *Yoga Nidra* is bringing you to a total physical and mental balance. Be aware of the consciousness within you. You are now feeling the energy flowing through your body and completely from point to point. Now you are becoming aware of your right hand, right thumb, ring finger, middle finger, index finger and the little finger. Feel the tips of the fingers. Be aware of your palms, the wrist, the elbow, the shoulders, the armpit, the right side of the trunk, the right thigh, the knee cap, the calf muscle, the ankle, the heel, the sole. Become aware of your right sole, the right foot, the right big toe, second toe, third toe, fourth toe and the fifth toe. Become aware of the left hand thumb, second finger, third finger, fourth finger and the little finger. Feel the tips of the fingers, left palm, left wrist, the elbow, the shoulder, the arm-pit and now, the left side of the trunk, the left thigh, the knee cap, the calf muscles, the ankle, the heel, the sole of the left foot, the big toe, second toe, third toe, fourth toe and fifth toe.

Now you are becoming aware of the top of the head. Both sides of the forehead, the right eye brow, the left eye brow, the space between the eye brows. Feel this particular psychic center very deeply. Become aware of the right ear, the left ear, the right cheek, the left cheek, the nose, the tip of the nose, the upper lip, the lower lip, the chin, the throat, the right side of the chest, the left side of the chest, the middle of the chest, the navel and the abdomen. Now you are becoming aware of your back. Become aware of the right shoulder blade, the left shoulder blade, the right buttock, the left buttock. Now stress your consciousness upon your spine from lower end to upper end and then over the whole of the back.

Now the awareness is pervading all the parts of the body, whole of right leg, whole of left leg. Both legs together, whole of right arm, whole of left arm, both arms together. whole of the back, buttocks, spine, whole of the front of abdomen, chest and the whole of the face... face... face.

The whole of the head together, the whole of the body together... your body is lying totally relaxed on the floor. You are seeing your body lying perfectly still on the floor in this room.

Now just become aware of your natural breathing. You are breathing in... breathing out... feel the flow of your breath in and out of your lungs... the rhythm of your breathing is natural, automatic. Now you are looking on the movements of your navel. It is rising and falling with every breath. Now start counting your breath from 21 to 0. Breathe in first keeping in mind the number 21 and breathe out keeping in mind the same number. Repeat this exercise every time diminishing the number by 1 till you reach zero. If you make a mistake go back to 21 and start all over again. Do not miss a single count... you are counting the breaths with your entire attention don't go to sleep... now, leave the counting at whatever the number you are and detach your awareness from your breathing.

Now you are recollecting the experience of pain, any kind of pain you have experienced in your life, remember the pain, feel that pain... now, try to experience the feeling of pleasure any pleasure remember the feeling of pleasure... now, again come back and feel yourself from head to toe to head.

Just feel a calm and quiet early morning. We are walking side by side on the bank of the river with clean and transparent water, both sides of the river are green, cool breeze is kissing our faces. The whole morning is splendid and beautiful, the birds are singing and now... you are alone just walking away from all the noise of the city. Now you are seeing the sun rise. It is like a crimson red ball, gradually coming up. Now you are feeling the divine pink rays emerging from the sun. They are entering into each and every part of your body. Your whole body is being merged in the divine light of pink rays. You are walking near a small place of worship on the bank. Now you are moving inside the temple... very calm... sitting softly there... with closed eyes, meditating deeply merging your consciousness with the super consciousness.

You are going in complete solitude and tranquillity. Inner bliss is flowing within you... now, remember your resolve that you made at the beginning of the *Yoga Nidra*. Repeat the same, resolve thrice with full awareness and strength... Gently come back from the inner journey to the surface again, back to your body. Become aware of your natural breathing. When you are aware give a slight movement to the body parts.

When you feel wide awake gently turn to the right, taking your own time; without hurry and slowly sit up calmly. Open your eyes. The *Yoga Nidra* has ended."

Around 1975, we came across transcendental meditation at the Ashram at Rishikesh. We were inducted into TM by a trained *guru*. He further inducted us into advanced TM techniques that are derived from *sutras* in Patanjali's *Yoga Sutra.*

We experienced the benefits for the stress removal. When we practiced TM meditation regularly, the benefits were self-evident. This was further revealed when we completed the treatment of a ruptured ectopic pregnancy, from diagnosis, admission, wheeling onto the operation table, exploratory laparotomy and blood transfusion within 18 minutes. Therefore, we decided to delve into different schools of meditation, as well as to study hypnotherapy in depth. Bihar School of Yoga was founded by Swami Satyanand

Saraswati. He used the term *Yoga Nidra* that was taught as a meditative practice. We have found that *Yoga Nidra* and meditation that was taught by Swami Chinmayananda, though differently named by different *gurus* are essentially the same. The metrics may differ, but substantially *Yoga Nidra* that now we equate as self hypnosis are basically the same with non-specific stress relief.

Alternatively, a hypnotherapist may treat any person with a new script. The guidelines for the script would be the personality, symptoms, belief system, etc. of the subject and motivation will be self improvement or getting rid of the symptoms/underlying causes.

Self Hypnosis—Visit to a garden

(For induction, refer to Self Hypnosis, Page. 84)

The relaxation wave is now gently spreading.

Now we are having a nice trip... would you like to have a nice trip with me? (ID; proceed only after Yes/No response). How nice... very nice... very intelligent... brilliant, why should you deny yourself a pleasure trip? Are you ready to go? (ID; proceed only after Yes/No response).

Now we are going out of this room... you see yourself getting up from the comfortable chair... remain seated... while you see yourself... getting up from the comfortable chair... remain seated... we are going out of this room... it has rained outside... there is pleasant co..o..l fre... sh... air as we go down the stairs... we are going out of this room... there is pleasant co..o..l fre... sh... air as we go down the stairs... Have we descended the stairs and are we out in the fresh and pleasant air? (ID; proceed only after Yes/No response). And, there, as we move on... as we move on... we arrive at...

...yourself... standing on the ground of a lovely house, enjoying the warm sun and the gentle breeze which fans your cheeks... breeze which fans your cheeks... (ID; proceed only after Yes/No response).

From this ground, you notice that there is a flight of ten steps leading down into a beautiful garden. Would you like that we go to the garden? (ID; proceed only after Yes/No response).

Go down these steps, one at a time,... one at a time,... linking your movement to an exhalation of your breath, feeling that, with each step you let go more and more. This sense of ever growing calm has completely enfolded you by the time you reach the garden. (ID: proceed only after Yes/No response).

And what a beautiful garden it is. You can see the masses of multi-coloured flowers, an ornamental fountain, superb shrubs, and graceful trees. There is V... i... b... g... y..o... r... white and black too! Perhaps you can smell the flowers, hear the songs of the birds, and the sound of the water from the fountain splashing into the pool at its base, and feel the gentle warmth of the sun soaking into your body. (ID; proceed only after Yes/No response).

Such wonder! Such delight! Such Joy! When you are enjoying... When you are enjoying... the time is running fast... the time is running fast... it is your natural due to... e... n... j... o... y... e... n... j... o... y. Let us... e... n... j... o... y as fast as we can... e... n... j... o... y time is just running out... it is but a few minutes... e... n... j... o... y is just running out... it is but a few minutes... but it is within your abilities... your highly hypnotic talents... to prolong the time... time can be prolonged... at your will... e... n... j... o... y... able...time can be so prolonged that you can enjoy this moment for a life time... A thing of beauty is joy for ever... (ID: proceed only after Yes/No response). That is your talent that life is getting happier... happier (ID; proceed only after Yes/No response) than your heart is just able to bear!

It is my privilege... trance is a great adventure and, highly intelligent and talented group that we are... we are... highly intelligent and talented group highly intelligent and talented people understand, yes... they understand what good suggestion is. Yes... you are... highly intelligent and talented... you understand what a good suggestion is. (ID; proceed only after Yes/No response).

And, I want you to go into a deeper and deeper state of trance... trance is to be calm, cool, composed... be calm, cool, composed and comfortable... completely relaxed... let go... to a state of natural innocence. Natural innocence of a baby like mind... curious and yet... innocent. Relax... Re... lax.

As you listen to my voice... As you listen to my voice... you relax even more. So much more that your eyelids are your own eyelids... (ID; proceed only after Yes/No response is elucidated). How wonderful to find... wonderful to find... that they have gone so heavy... heavy... that they are getting heavier and more heavier... that they are like lead curtains... wonderful to find... more heavier... like lead curtains... so that you are not able to open them... more heavier... try to open them and... find that you are not able to open them...

Keep taking a deep... deeper and deeper breath and as you do so... as you are doing so... you go into a deeper and deeper state of trance... and you find that your right hand... your right hand is getting lighter and lighter... lighter than air... it goes up in the air... yes, it is going up in the air... up and up and up... slowly,... slowly,... slowly,... but surely see that it is going up in the air, how wonderful to be able to see with your closed eyes... yes, it is going up in the air... up and up and up... And, now that it has gone up... it stays there. No weight in your arm... lighter and lighter... lighter than air... (ID; proceed only after Yes/No response).

Self Hypnosis

The number in brackets represents repetition in the script delivery.

The subject is introduced to the Mind which can gather new knowledge, new experience, new wisdom. In the 4th state/trance mind will be calm and peaceful and not interfere.

"Take a Comfortable position. Allow your whole body to become loose (3) when you feel totally relaxed (3). With your close eyes I want to see your whole body relaxed and resting peacefully. Observe your whole body from top of your head to foot (each part being described) and see how your mental eyes see your body resting peacefully, relaxed and feeling cool, and quiet. If you want to make yourself to be comfortable you can move any part of your body Rest in more comfortable position you are free to move and more comfortable position. Check, recheck (2).

Mind has learnt new knowledge, new experience, new wisdom. Soft sponge absorbs all liquids poured on, it relax comfortably and resting and respond to this session of mind. Your mental self has seen your whole self at peace created within you, created in your physical body.

Watch your spontaneous breathing. The chest wall, the abdomen wall is moving spontaneously, rhythmically, continuously. All are bringing about a vital activity of nature. You are able to observe the nurture that occurs in you. It happens due to exchange of gases. It happens regularly, repeatedly, rhythmically without your knowledge. May be feeling your breathing process or sensing your breathing process you are now fully absorbed in attending your breathing process. Man by observing nature has learnt many lessons. Being a product of nature may be nature creates new things. Nature's universal law of breathing for survival is going on in you through your breathing process. As you watch your breathing process, which is a dynamic activity, you find every breath you take in you take fresh air. With every breath out you are throwing out impure air, in life also all impure materials, thoughts, habit, mind programme has to be discarded for new ideas, feelings, sensations to come in.

As you watch your breathing process, you find your lungs expand to receive fresh air. Likewise your mind enjoys learning, new learnings. New wisdom, new knowledge, new experience, joy, new life enhancing thoughts. See now as your lungs are experiencing to receive fresh air, the same way your mind also is expanding experiencing, enlarges, enlightens to receive new learning of knowledge, new wisdom and experience new joy with each breath in. After exchange of gases you find your lungs squeeze impure air, out of your respiratory tract through your nose. This action of the lungs to squeeze the impure air out is an activity of nature. It shows that what has been used, its utility served has to be discarded. The remaining part if it remains, it has toxic effect on the body system.

Has to be emptied. The lung squeezing out the impure air, the used air, the old air, is now making you realize that in mind also whatever is not required for your present and future utility has to be thrown out. But stored in the past, may be knowingly or unknowingly, is to be removed. So I want you to remove all unwanted things to be removed with each breath out throwaway all your sad feelings, all negative thoughts, bad memories, all your hatred, all your jealousy, selfishness and lastly all your guilt. Remove it. Throw it out.(3)

See how nature has its own way to make you understand nature's wisdom.

As you watch your breathing process, as you throw out impure air, I want you to throw out all your sad feelings etc., all your guilt, knowingly or unknowingly been the victim to circumstances. And reacting impulsively, to make things, to make events, to make feelings worst for you. Remove it, throw it out as lungs throw out impure air make space for new air to come in, I want you to realize that you have made enough space for new thoughts, creative ideas, more space in your mind by discarding, emptying, removing all your anger, hatred etc. and finally all your guilt. REMOVE IT THROW IT OUT ----(3)

See how you start working and cleaning your mind from outside in, your outer mind or conscious mind. Then I want you to go into inner mind or your subconscious mind and unconscious mind and remove all your sad feelings, bad memories, your frustration, all your anger sometimes towards yourself the anger and sometimes anger, displeasure to your near and dear ones, Remove it for your generosity to forgive yourself. Throw away selfishness etc.

May be your inner mind to be cleaned it up, I want you to go back in age to go back in time 2009—8—7—5—4—3—2—1-2000, 1994-1770—1659—go back in time to your past life to many past life, for your mind and being eternal, passing from life to life thereby having continuity but today realizing that your mind is to be cleaned, mind is to be transformed, I want you to clean your mind and throw away from your mind all negative thoughts etc. from your personal life, professional life, all related to the past, throw it out. As anything that stagnates it always stinks. Do not want you to see or experience your past which is not useful to you. SO CLEAN YOUR MIND from all your past which knowingly or unknowingly been photographed and preserved in your memory bank in your mind, remove it throw it out.

See how your whole mind is being cleaned by you and yourself. It involves mental effort. It is a difficult process. Though it is difficult it feels clean, nice, shining, mental commitment, mental determination, but I want you to throw away inner mind, empty out all your sad feelings etc. and lastly your guilt.

To persist in your effort, and persevere in your determination, I want you to dig in your inner mind from side to side. Top to bottom, in and out, up and down, going back in age, going back in time, you are cleaning your inner mind, your unconscious mind, all your sad feelings etc

You deserve a healthy body and healthy mind. A healthy mind in a healthy body. A healthy mind working constructively, creatively to make you have positive thoughts, enjoy your life in the present. Make goal in life, a vision to succeed and make you aware of the prosperity and world showing you are achieving by loving yourself and gifting yourself your own love. You are making yourself an important person, responsible person happy through your mind. See how we who should change, it is I who should change, it is I who is responsible, it is I who am, and my happiness depends on the love I pour to myself, I give to myself. I owe to myself. From now onwards, I love myself, from this moment I make myself happy, to make me successful, make me prosperous, fulfil all my dreams. See how like flower blooming from a bud according to nature's love you have transformed yourself to most beautiful flower unknowingly spreading its fragrance to its surroundings. You are a gifted person chosen by God to your own responsibility, to yourself through your mind. As you work on it, you will materialize God's plan for you to realize the closeness to yourself and to the inner God within you. Inner god, philosopher, guide, friend, protector is within you. You are complete and have independent identity, inner purity, and inner beauty you rightly deserve. It is up to you to be aware of yourself, through this relaxation session, it takes time, your effort but with your determination, dedication, passion, persistence, you are conquering your own happiness, joy in life, to succeed in life and to become prosperous achieve high set goal in life. See how God plans everything, designs everything in your favour gives you abundant opportunity, to realize your purpose in life. See how knowingly or unknowingly all the obstacles you are facing have influenced your thinking to give you the experience, knowledge, wisdom, you have achieved with your struggle. Now utilizing that wisdom, experience to mature yourself and grow rich in your mind. I want you to think positively, constructively, creatively apply this experience to make you happy person, healthy person, and successful person in life. See how you deserve to fertilize the soil to work on it with determination, dedication, and persistence to prepare a fertile soil, to swathe seed that it grows a healthy plant, you are working through your mind to fertilize your mind outer mind and inner mind make it healthy, wealthy, creative, constructive to make yourself a happy person in life.

As you watch your breathing process, being in a relaxed state, it establishes oneness with the universal consciousness, union of consciousness.

Nature is providing you with abundant wisdom, knowledge, opportunity, power, to be creative constructive to live a healthy, happy life with full of spirituality. See how you are working with your mind to change your life, to transfer your life, to so appropriate seed to grow healthy plant, healthy tree, produce flowers, fruits so that it spreads fragrance everywhere in environment which nature appreciates, acknowledges and also glorifies, is proud to possess you are the creator of your joy, success prosperity and wealth. You deserve happiness, joy, God's child, to be nature's child. You deserve to be communicated to be wise, knowledgeable, and give you strength to conquer and convert your weaknesses to strength to make you prosperous in life. Your nourished mind, your nurtured mind, your fertilised mind is now transferring your mind to make you happy, to make you healthy and to make you come over all the weaknesses and obstacles in life. Now gathering all this beautiful memories I want you to come back to yourself slowly become fully aware, when you feel like come back to full awareness and become alert and awake.

Enjoy inner harmony, joy, stillness and quietness.

Your mind has sensed peace, inner joy in your whole body. Whole mind is attending your breathing process, so spontaneous thoughts are passing by, spontaneous thoughts are becoming lesser, lesser and lesser and you are likely to start experiencing trance. So the thoughts are becoming lesser, lesser and thoughts are disappearing. As they are disappearing you are going in to trance.

Vital activity of nature and nurture by you which occurs regularly rhythmically seeing your breathing process, taking fresh air. You are throwing out impure air, impure thoughts, unwanted feelings, New knowledge, new joy, life enhancing experience are expanding, experience squeezing action of lungs. Its action is to squeeze.

The mind has sad feelings, all your frustration, bad feelings jealousy, all your guilt knowingly or unknowingly making all your bad memories, all your anger, selfishness, negative thoughts. It is Nature's wisdom, each breath you take you remove used air, as you start working on cleaning your outer mind or conscious mind. Remove from your inner mind anger. The anger on yourself or on your near ones or dear ones is harming everybody. So remove it. From your broad mind or heart, or due to your generosity, throw away all bad memories, etc.

From your memory, your photographic memory, remove all unwanted thoughts, all bad memory, all ill feelings is thrown out.

Age regression 2009—2008—2007—2006—2000—1900—1700—700—-Feeling the eternal self, the soul being ever present.

You are experiencing universal energy, divine energy. You are confident, comfortable, concentrating, and courageous.

Throw out sad feeling, bad memory, all frustrations, negative thoughts, ill feelings, jealousy, selfishness, and lastly all your guilt. Remove it, throw it out, clean it out, clear out your system completely.

Let your mind and body is free of it. Continue to do it through your breathing activity."

Stress Relief—Controlling 5 senses—Garden, feeling of breeze, singing birds, sunrise, fragrance of flowers, sweet taste in mouth

For induction refer to page 84.

And as I'm so relaxed that in this relaxation position I open the door, go down the stairs and I come in the front of Sayaji Garden and stand there in this relaxed position and ready to walk, ready to walk in the garden. It's 9th of January, it's about the dawn is ending and the morning is about to begin it is 7 o' clock. The doors are open. I'm listening various birds singing, answering in their own language and a fine breeze touches my cheeks. It is very, very soothing, feel very happy with the touch and with that touch the fragrance of the flower that is there on the side, a small bush on either side near the pavement. I am experiencing this favourite, my favourite fragrance and I stand there for a few seconds to visualize these beautiful colours of the flowers and enjoy this beautiful fragrance, a cool breeze and I move forward. I have come to this garden many times but today I'm listening this music experiencing the whole peaceful, tranquil, early morning atmosphere and walk onward enjoying the whole atmosphere and as I walk I see a small pond at a distance and I want to experience which I am seeing is a Lotus pond. I walk little faster and come near this Lotus pond and I am seeing various colours of lotuses. They are white like a white swan. They had a pink shade and they are blue.

I just stand there and as the breeze flows, few water droplets move on the leaves of these beautiful flowers and they are dancing like small transparent beads but does not wet the surface. They keep on dancing going to and fro and make various shapes and again they dissolve. As I'm watching these droplets dancing, I have brought some peanuts. With the smell of this peanut as I'm watching these droplets I see various colour of fish coming up on the surface watching me and my hand. I pick up a few groundnuts and throw into the water and this fish 1, 2, 3, they jump; take this and just disappear and again more fish come up the surface and I see this beautiful dance of nature. The droplets dancing on the leaves, the breeze mildly make the Lotus flower dance and the fish come on the surface takes away the groundnut and I can see it opening the mouth swallowing and disappear. As I'm watching and enjoying this dance of nature, the quiet communion in consciousness, I just see at the horizon. It is a beautiful, wonderful, quiet, cool situation. The whole panorama gradually on the Far East, I see a beautiful red slit gradually moving up and up and from slit it becomes 1/3 of a circle and half and gradually that is a red ball changing its colour and it is a beautiful sunrise. I am just wonderstruck extremely happy dancing within myself as I'm watching. I had watched a Crimson red is changing its colour and as it comes up it loses its red dress and becoming lighter and lighter and it becomes yellow, I'm very happy to be here. I have enjoyed and all my worries, all my tensions have disappeared. There is so much of pleasure in my mind and in my brain that I love this wonderful spiritual experience in the space that I have created in my brain and made become a part of me. I'm sitting down on a bench to experience this moment of joy, happiness, and tranquillity of self.

Stress Relief—Flying in the clouds

For induction refer to page 84.

You are sitting on a bench in the garden, while I see up a white fluffy cloud in front of this yellow bright sun in the light is little bit obstructed but I keep on and enjoying this change in the atmosphere and this white fluffy cloud becomes a little darker and darker and I feel like flying in this cloud and I am part of this cloud. And I am flying in this beautiful atmosphere and this fluffy cloud turns darker and becomes still darker and gets filled up with moisture and it is black and it starts raining. I am flying in this cloud and the water droplets fall on me and I feel very very cool. It makes me wet and the water passes from my back and falls on the ground and gradually the cloud again reappears white and disappears and I come back on the ground and there is a small stream of water flowing and on the bank of that stream. I FEEL COOL, COMFORTABLE AND STRESS FREE.

Experience of Meditation

(Devi Durga can be changed according to the belief system)

I am sitting by a gentle stream and there is a small temple of Devi Durga with 18 hands having all the equipments of various kinds in all her 18 hands. I find them very, very useful and the *aarti* begins. I sit on the footsteps of the temple putting my legs in the stream which is very cool, comfortable and become one with this divine spiritual atmosphere of nature for few seconds.

Now *aarti* is finished, I with folded hands, bow down to this wonderful, beautiful experience that I have enjoyed fully. Sit quietly for few seconds and having enjoyed, having put this full experience in myself. Having thrown away all the stresses, all the anxiety and feeling fine, fresh energized. I am gradually waking up telling myself all the time feeling very relaxed but at the same time very energized with full determination of getting back home to start my morning. I am fully energized, confident self and I am walking back out of the garden.

Terminate the trance.

Cleaning up the room—(Mind)

For induction, refer to page 84.

I have a room which is not been opened since long and it is having furniture. It is studded with old furniture. Some broken and others can be used. As a child, I remember a nice cupboard, which on entering the room I can see lying in the corner. The whole room is full of dust. As I try to enter, I start taking out the furniture one by one. Chairs, tables, small cupboards, intact or broken. I take it out one by one and make into two rows—one intact and other broken. I continuously keep on cleaning the room to go near the cupboard with a nice Belgian mirror where I can see myself! But at one corner there is a big black blot which I am not able to clean with the ordinary or wet cloth. I have brought a chemical which can clean up any stain. I take it on a piece of cloth and start cleaning. It is very deep rooted and as I rub it hard, at a corner I see it is disappearing. I am very happy that I have made it and so I clean up the whole blot and I see in front of the mirror, myself, absolutely clean, shining, clear and stress free. Yes, I have made it!

Walking through the forest—Stress relief

For induction, refer to page 84.

I am walking on a path with a river flowing by my side and on either side there are tall trees, birds singing and time of sunrise. At a distance I see a forest with tall trees of various kinds and shrubs but it is very dark. Suddenly I come near the entrance and I find a stick. Hardly I can see the path, I have a torch and I try to enter. So many shrubs and small plants have intermingled and with the stick which is very strong in my hand I make my path which is very narrow. I am gradually moving forward to reach the other end of the forest. The river flowing by my side is my guideline and I am able to make my way with the help of the stick and suddenly at a distance, I see a ray of sun entering into this dark forest and I realize that I have made it. I move forward and come to the end of the forest, happy, joyful and being successful I stand in front of the sun which is become yellow and above the horizon. I feel like dancing with joy, tranquillity, peace and happiness. Yes, I have made it!"

Another demonstration of hypnotherapeutic phenomena is hypnoanaesthesia

Krishna Joshi, a physiotherapist, joined the training course for hypnotherapy. She volunteered to demonstrate hypnoanaesthesia. This was even transferred to one side of the cheek. This was photographed and is illustrated in the second part of this book.

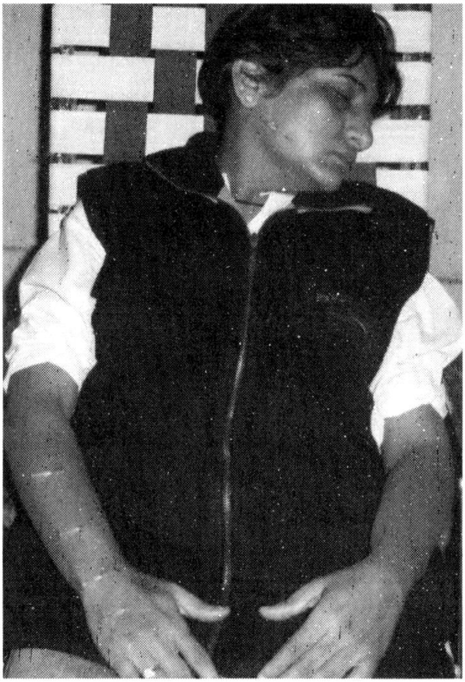

Hypnoanaesthesia with picture of needles in forearm and transfer to cheek.

This buttressed her belief that hypnotherapy must be a science though some of the phenomena like absence of pain and its transfer to other parts of the body remains unexplained scientifically. We treated her teenage niece, Khushboo, with Amyotrophic Lateral Sclerosis, also an autoimmune disorder. We were delighted a few years later to see the patient, the niece, treating physiotherapy patients as per the instruction by Krishna Joshi. After few years, physiotherapist Krishna herself suffered from systemic lupus erythematosus. It is an autoimmune disease in which the immune system attacks its own tissues, causing widespread inflammation and tissue damage in the affected organs. However, the patient Krishna this time had profound faith in hypnotherapy. As soon as she realized the symptoms, she started to get up in the morning at 04:30, walk down to the temple which is about 3 km away and walk back home with continuous chanting of Lord Krishna—Vasudeva and later on for an hour, she would sit for meditation. With positive assertion that every particle of food that she swallows is a remedy sent to her by Lord Krishna—Vasudeva. She excluded all nocebos.

All the time that she is awake, there will be a continuous background chanting of various *mantras*. It has created a pious atmosphere in her clinic and at her home. This has not only helped her but also the subjects attending her clinic. A doctor friend just visits the clinic to experience the ambience and goes into trance.

She in now without any symptoms of SLE and treating with physiotherapy her patients at her clinic!

Suggestion for Pain—Ice tray

For induction refer to page 84.

You are now seeing a gorgeous mansion. There are sprawling lawns and beautiful gardens around the building. You are walking up to your own home... and with each step into the mansion, it lights up from basement to the attic (ID; proceed only after Yes/No response is elucidated). It is your own house... your own home... home sweet home... home is where heart is... and you have entered the kitchen in your own house where every day... every day you eat nutritious food and drink cold... .cold, chilled water... refreshing chilled water with ice. You are walking up to the refrigerator... and now you have opened the fridge and... a cold breeze envelop you... as the refrigerator is open. Open the eyes compartment with your right/left hand... and you have taken out the ice trays... and you have taken out the ice trays. (ID; proceed only after Yes/No response). You are taking out the ice cubes one by one by one by one by one... and your hand your right/left hand is getting cold and numb... and it is... it is absolutely numb and frozen. Yes it is frozen ice... absolutely numb no sensation all the way no sensation all the way up to elbow. Your hand is numb, absolutely numb, no sensation up to the elbow... frozen ice.

Terminate the trance with the arm up to elbow staying anaesthetized.

Results

At the end of the session 23/27 subjects experienced 3rd stage of hypnosis. A second sample of blood, 2 ml was withdrawn. 23/27 did not feel the pain of 2nd prick. A post-session interview by the hypnotherapist in-charge was conducted to verify the depth of hypnosis utilizing the following criteria:

1. Experience fragrance of perfume.
2. Felt descending steps.
3. Felt warm breeze on cheek.
4. Experience time being extended.
5. Eyelids get heavier.
6. Hand go up in air.
7. Experience anaesthesia.

Stress/Relaxation Session

Using a variety of metaphors like:

- **Barrenness/Desert**
- **Third Eye**
- **Alice in Wonderland**
- **Roses/Garden**

Welcome... Welcome my friends... Both of you are welcome to a session. A session that I promise you. I promise you once again that this session is so powerful and it is so designed so as it can entirely... it will entirely change... I promise that it will entirely change your life.

The life will so change that in there is so much of sand (3)... and barrenness. Barrenness is like a desert and even in this desert land, today you are now relaxing and take a deep, deep, and deep breath... As you take a deep, a deep, and deeper breath,... relax... relax... relax all the muscles of your body. Relaxation is a natural state, natural state is where the comfort is and you are feeling. Now with each breath you take, and you have taken a deeper and deeper breath, take a deep, deep, deep breath. And while that deep breath has relaxed you, slowly let it go. With each breath getting out, so much carbon dioxide is, so much carbon dioxide, as you know, is getting out of your system and carbon dioxide is not good, while oxygen is life.

So, take once again a deep and deeper breath and see how you have found yourself so relaxed that your eyelids. Your right and left eyelids are... both the eyelids are... both the eyelids are drooping down... it is getting more and more difficult to keep your eyes open. And yet if you like to keep your eyes open... if you like to keep your eyes open, you may keep them open... and as you decide, you find that closing the eyes is so much better for you to relax... when we close our eyes... when we close our eyes, we not only close, we tend to close the impulses, the visual impulses from outside world and when the visual impulses from outside world are no more received... no more received by the brain, the brain... the brain opens. The brain opens a third eye. The third eye... the inner eye... the eye of perception... P. E. R. C. E. P. T. I. O. N... this third eye is a natural gift given by Nature to all human beings but so far you have not even known yourself and opening of the third eye is like... the opening of the third eye is like the first step of Alice in Wonderland. Now, you are seeing yourself... yourself, so daintily dressed, so pretty and so much full of joy that Alice is so happy to have entered... Alice is so happy to have entered the land of Wonderland and this wonderland that always... was always... and is always there with us, barely we have had... barely we have had a glimpse of this. But this wonderland is so full... so full of beauty, wonder, joy and so much of profound astonishment... profound... P. R. O. F. O. U. N. D astonishment that is also apart from being a Wonderland, it happens... it happens to be the land... it happens to be the land of wish fulfilment. Have you any particular wish? Think of that wish and see... see for yourself, even advancing yourself in time that in a naturally allocated time that your wish is fulfilled... This is the beauty of this Wonderland... this is the beauty of this land of wish fulfilment and there are several other unknown, so far to you... unknown so far to you, several occurrences... the world itself has changed... the world has so changed that there is only beauty... there is everything is so nice and everything that happens is as per your wish. So, when you feel that the Alice has seen the beautiful world full of roses, and roses of all colours! There are roses (3) in this garden and when you see a garden full of roses of all colours move... move index finger of your right hand. When you move the index finger of the right hand, I know that you have... that you have seen a rose garden and the rose garden is full of... rose garden is full of roses of all colours. See for yourself, there is a usual colour for a rose... the usual colour for the rose is pink and you are seeing a courtyard... you have seen a courtyard that is full of pink and various shades of red roses... and as you feel happy... and please... Oh, such beautiful roses and all of them are there in my garden... I must, must feel happy at this moment. And as now we both feel happy, you move index finger of your right hand...

Thank you. Thank you. And when you want to see only and only... when you want to see more beautiful roses, move the index finger of your right hand... take your time... they are definitely there are what your open eyes have not been able to see before, the inner eye... inner eye that sees truth, beauty and joy... the inner eye that sees truth, beauty and joy. And truth, beauty and joy are best seen as personified... personified truth, beauty and joy are seen with various shades of flowers... now your inner eye... your inner eye has seen a violet flower... maybe it is a rose, maybe it is a variant of rose... but flower that surely is and what a beautiful violet flower. Would you like to see... even more beauty... how the life can be much more beautiful and when beauty is beautiful, why should you hesitate to see it. Say yes... say yes by moving the index finger of your right hand. And there as you have said yes, your partner who has come with you has also closed the eyes and has joined you in this Wonderland... your friend has also joined with closing the eyes and taking deep and deeper breaths and he has to catch up with you and there it is... the eyes of your partner are also closed and both of them... you that are there like little children in that garden... garden of Alice in Wonderland... and so nice to see the whole spectrum of flowerbeds... they are blue... you saw the violet flower, we are now seeing blue... the rare kind of blue roses and they are also interspersed with indigo... the indigo roses are so wonderful, so rare... your garden is full of violet, indigo, blue roses... see them... feel joy and beauty and that time move the index finger of your right hand... Thank you. This wonderful experience is so wonderful that we can change not only the colours of the flowers but we can change the pattern of arrangement and the flowers of whatever kind and you can also choose... you can also choose... let us choose the kind of most favourite fragrance... choose... choose most favourite fragrance and as you take a further deep breath, how wonderful! What an accomplishment... what a latent power... latent power of your mind that you have now mastered to... you have mastered to bring into manifestation... you have mastered and experienced the mastery of your mind... feel a fine fragrance... deep, deeper and deeper breath... and when you and your friend take a deep breath together, then it gets easier so take a deep, deep, and deep breath and feel the fragrance... feel the fragrance... favourite fragrance of your choice... and as you feel the favourite fragrance, please move any of the fingers of your right hand... Thank you. And this fine fragrance is the fragrance of your choice so why not have it with you for the entire day today? Would you like that this fragrance, fine, favourite fragrance of your choice stays with you for the whole day today? If yes, say yes by moving your right index finger... Take your time... But why deny... why deny a natural occurrence that is available to you simply with a master manifestation... manipulation so simple that you can have the fragrance now or it will persist even after the session or it may persist for the rest of the day... You need not share with me what is your choice... But please make a choice of the perfume and gently write it down in the memory of this present moment.

We have travelled a long distance from the everyday world where most of the times we are not... most of the time in the everyday life, we are not the master of our mind. That we have unfortunately accepted by not understanding the power... the power... the power that is given to our minds by mother Nature. Mother Nature has made every human being a master of himself or herself and now that you have seen the power that your mind has, it has been my privilege to have shared this moment where I myself have been with you in this Alice that we all turned ourselves into in this world of Wonderland. I thank you... Thank you when we meet again.

When a hypnotherapist induces trance, the state is akin to *Turya*. When a therapist teaches self hypnosis to a patient or even a healthy subject, the difference between self hypnosis and *Yoga Nidra* disappears. The difference remains only in the mind of the practitioner.

Group Hypnosis

Hypnosis is an experiential phenomena. In group hypnosis, the participants who do not want to be put into trance and only observe are asked to sit on the left (It automatically becomes a shift of paradigm). In our experience, those who are wanting to observe go into trance earlier than the other participants. Those who resist are often affected with minor symptoms like headache, backache, or pain in the neck. At the end of the session, these participants are relieved by putting them back into trance for few minutes and woken up.

The subjects are put into a trance by PMR and deep breathing. The complaints were backache, resistant nasal discharge, wanting to be a *Braj Gopi*, etc. The suggestions began with common suggestions for ego strengthening and stress reduction. The therapists then went from subject to subject, giving suggestions specific to the complaints expressed by the subjects. When the subject given suggestions for a specific complaint, the rest of the participants were asked to be in deep trance so as to not listen to any other discussion going on.

Yoga Nidra—1st session (Group Hypnosis)

History of the subject: Anu was a lady of 30 years, unmarried,

Krishna *bhakt*[1], wanted to be a *Braj Gopi*. The family wanted her to be settled in married life. She was going from pillar to post and finally joined the Ashram in Prashanti, Bangalore. She volunteered for hypnotherapy and past life regression reach to her aim to be *Krishna bhakt*. Below is the first session of *Yoga Nidra* that she was made to experience in a group hypnosis setting.

(Addressing the name of the subject say Anu in this session)

Anu, please take a comfortable position in the chair. Yes very nice. Take a deep breath in and out, wonderful and as you are taking a deep breath in and out, you can wriggle your toes and move your hand and finger, so that you remove all the tension from the body and throw it out of the system. You start relaxing from the soul of your feet, wonderful, yes, very nice. Let all the tension go out and relax. Relaxation wave is gradually moving up and up, it goes to both ankle and also both the legs. It moves up to both the knees. There are tendons which are supporting the knees and also fibrous strands which are working continuously supporting the knees. It helps in walking, standing and also in keeping you steady all the time. Just let them relax. The thighs have bulky muscles in front and back. They are enjoying this relaxation. So the blood flows to and fro in this relax state. All the time getting fresh blood and throwing out all the rubbish it makes those bulky muscles feel loose, light. There is space between the fibers with free blood flow. It makes it energized, relaxed and quiet.

The wave of this energized relaxation is moving upward to make front and back of the abdomen relaxed, cool and comfortable. As the coolness enters through the abdominal wall, all the organs in the abdomen gets vitalized by the fresh oxygenated blood and feels fresh, energized and also tranquil, peaceful and quiet. It moves forward towards chest. You can experience your breathing getting quiet, peaceful and harmonious. The heart is beating regularly and slowly but with great vigour. The shoulder, arms and palm of the hand is cool and comfortable. The fingers of the hand can be moved if you like. But due to feeling absolutely free of tension if you like, you can just enjoy that deep relaxation. Along the neck it is moving slowly to the facial muscles. They are small and fine muscles. When they relax, your whole face relaxes. That relaxed, magnificent smile of your face makes you look 10 years younger. That smile of yours is wonderful.

As it enters your head, the mind is enjoying this state of trance and also the whole brain is feeling happy. Keep enjoying this trance of happiness.

> "I am feeling relaxed, happy, tranquil all over myself, very, very quiet, enjoying this state of happiness, this state of being, cool, comfortable and now I would like to move forward".

I am moving out from the room of Prashanti of and going out to a place of my choice. I am there and it is just before the sun rise. The darkness of night is just disappearing and first ray of light is seen at the horizon on the east. The atmosphere is beautiful. There are big trees and plenty of colourful flower beds. There is fine fragrance of various flowers and it is feeling up the whole surrounding as well as my whole self. The birds are waking up with their biological clock. They are hopping up from one branch to other. They are chirping and also calling their mate. That symphony is so nicely tuned. It really pleases my ears. The cool, fine breeze is passing through the leaves and also is spreading fine mixed fragrance all around me. It touches my face and makes me feel very happy. I am enjoying this surrounding with all its contents.

In a short while the east horizon is changing its colour. I see a red streak which gradually rises up and moving forward to become a red ball of fire—The sun. Gradually with the majestic walk it moves upwards into the sky. It gives light all over the place without any discrimination. It enlightens all the people, rich or poor, young or old, healthy or sick!!!!!

How gorgeous!!! Like mother' love. Knows only to give without any expectation, any condition. Sun gives for the happiness to others. It gives light, cosmic energy unconditionally. Whoever wants it, they take it. What a virtue!!! It all depends on the individual who takes. But if one surrenders to the ALMIGHTY'S wish, then you have no exertion, no tension and just float like a bird. You have given away the reins in his hand. The almighty floats in the right direction. (just as Arjun gave chariot's control to lord Krishna).

The sun is gradually on its journey in the sky, moves higher and simultaneously and gradually from crimson red it has changed its colour to yellow. It is getting hot also. As I turn, I see nice temple. It has tall, nicely caved with various deities sculptures with pleasant features; it makes me feel very happy. As I enter the temple, it is time for *Arti*[2]. I hear the bells ringing and it makes familiar sound. It gives the primordial sound of AUM. There are many bells. They all are tuned in a symphony of morning tune. There is one bell as if left for me. I go and join in this symphony of bells. It fills up my self with immense joy, relaxation, peace, tranquillity. I go into trance and become one with the universal consciousness. I am in deep trance. This experience of being aware of everything has taken me away to the higher state of consciousness. This experience is beyond language. It is Ecstasy!!!! It is beyond verbal description. I want to feel up this experience in my heart and head. At any and every time of my need I want this experience to come handy to me.

Arti is over. I stand in front of the deity. As I stand there in front, I see the expression of welcome in the eyes of the deity. It makes me so happy. There are tears of joy rolling over my cheeks. I am absolutely steady as if I have become a statue. I stand with folded hands. The blessings are being showered. I am being blessed everyday but today's experience is completely new. I continue in this state of trance. It makes me feel peaceful from within. Not only that but I am in different state of CONSCIOUNESS. I am part of UNIVERSAL Consciousness. I am one with THEE. I feel very, very privileged, special, and happy. I want the place of this experience in my heart to last forever. I continue to be in this state till it integrates in me.(to be in this state for at least few minutes).

Suddenly I realize that so much of the time has passed. I wake up and birds are flying away for their daily routine leaving their little ones in the nest.

Trance can be terminated at this point for self hypnosis only. Further work can be continued for therapeutic session after this point depending on the complaint for up to 90 minutes.

Spirituality can be utilized for mental disorder, for better focus and memory enhancement and self-confidence.

(1) I also feel like flying in the sky. I take over to fly. I feel very, very light, (2) I am in the air. I am entering in to those woolly white clouds. The bright sun which had become hot is not seen. Oh! Where it has disappeared? Can the clouds cover the sun over? It is an illusion. I feel fine, enjoyable. These fine white woolly clouds change their colour and become brown and ultimately black. They are so heavy that they are unable to float. It turns into shower. As the droplets of water fall on me I enjoy every bit of it. Again I feel very light, energetic, and joyful. I see the cloud disappearing. I am able to float without any resistance. The sun is shining again with the same glory. It makes me feel happy, peaceful, light in my self, and tranquil. I feel very, very light, energetic, and joyful. All my tension and worries are gone.

I am flying like a carefree bird in the sky, flying for the joy of it, for the happiness and for the pleasure of it. I try to see up in the sky. I only see clear blue sky, brightly illumined, clear like crystal. As I try to see below, I see roads, car moving on it, small row of houses and big gardens from where I had taken this journey. I have achieved and gathered a fortune from this flight. I feel assured, confident, cool, comfortable and fully assured about my capabilities. I am convinced that I can perform what I am capable of doing. I am a free bird without any load on myself. On this journey, I happened to meet Dr. Vyas (Name of the therapist). He is happy to be flying with me. As I am flying higher and higher, I realize that I am made of a different stuff. I am so unique, special, singular, and specific. The nature, Mother nature has crafted me, sculpted me, designed me to excel in my own unique way in whatever that I wish to undertake to do. I shall undertake only such things that are noble, unique, magnificent, wonderful and excellent.

Be it a Sunday job of routine cleaning of my house or washing of my clothes, or studies (depending on the client's need, the suggestions are given) or excelling in the work of my duty or hobby or of choice, or even wanting to climb Mount Everest, I am made to excel in my own way and if excellence is myself, I am excellent, magnificent, I am wonderful.

My name is excellent incarnate and I will be excelling in my own way, I have shed inhibitions, reservations, and restrictions. My name is excellence itself. That excellence which is signified and symbolized in the feminine form of Saraswati, Vigneshwari, Jigneshwari, Vijayalaxmi, Maha Durga, Maha Kali is giving me help, guidance and showing me the way to act. (These are various forms of feminine consciousness). There is submergence of these Feminine excellences in myself. I want to supremely sublimate myself to a greater height of being a human being and in realizing the potential of flying high.

I have incorporated with in my flying high, the flying spirit of high riding Subramanian (Kartikeya, male energizing form). I am as capable as Kartikeya when he goes round the whole world like the bright shining sun, I also can go around the world, the universe. Totally convinced that masculinity is the valour and vigour of Kartikeya who excels in ardent pursuit of adventure and in so doing create many fold forms that is fine and beautiful.

With all the deities' help as Durga is powerful to reach her aim, I am powered by all these deities to reach my aim to become *Braj Gopi* and be like Mirabai or Narsinh Mehta.

(The trance was then terminated in a routine fashion and after couple of days she was a volunteer for past life regression)

From the complaints and symptoms, the therapist will arrive at the diagnosis and also the therapeutic strategy. The causes are more in unconscious mind which are tackled during the session. In Hypnosis some analysis occurs.

Following the session for 1 and half hour, she went into deep hypnosis and for 3 days, she was under observation with the attendant. She was fed and her daily routine was looked after by the attendant and when she woke up, all her myths and misconceptions were solved and had a long dialogue with the therapist.

Experience of Spirituality. (Anu in group hypnosis)

There is an Anupam (extra ordinary) experience. Anupama, Anu, (Atom), The me, The Anupama, there is no such other person than me that is Anupama, no comparable, my highly spiritual motivated self. This is natural due, I wanted, I aspired. My aspiration is noble to see God face to face, living incarnate, my physical self. As ANUPAMA is there, there is no second, there is union with Thee, there is no duality. I have merged into cosmic consciousness. I The Anu (Atom) can become so small and merge in to universe. And also pervade all over the sky and universe as universal consciousness. Now I know what it is to be with God. Let there be silence, as I go to highly sublime state of tranquillity, peace, beauty, and Beasts!!!! Where is the beast here? Beauty is beautiful by itself. A thing of beauty is joy forever. A beautiful state is truly blissful.

In Group Hypnosis, Komal (Delicate, tender) had backache.

Let Komal climb the Everest. She is climbing step by step(2). But me the Komal have a quantum jump. Yes I can take step by step and also, I the Komal, delicate Komal, wonderful Komal have set the foot on Mount Everest. I am jumping here.

Post Hypnotic suggestion

I shall be able to experience this any time and every time that I want to. I will listen to the recorded cassette, also it is recorded in my mind, this is a promise to myself that shall be fulfilled.

Discussion on age regression in absence of subject

Usually in age regression, the patient is taken very, very deep that takes much longer and also remains hypnoidal for a day or two. In case of Anu she remained sleeping for 48 hours and was hypnoidal for almost 3 days.

Q. If subject is forcefully woken up, what happens?

A. Psycho dynamically her work goes on, She is in trance, in such situation she is made comfortable. She is made to sleep and supervision is kept. Do not ever forcefully wake the subject up.

There is dual experience. Therapist is giving such intent session, then likely that he is also hypnoidal. So always process slowly, deliberately and in a focalized manner.

Q. Why take signature?

A. As one grows in age, the handwriting and the medium of communication changes. So from mother tongue to English and so on.

Past Life Regression

Ancient Indian tradition is fundamentally based on Hinduism and Buddhism. Even when Shankaracharya wrote his conclusive poem as *Bhajagovindam*, he reiterated that rebirth and further rebirth is going to propel the human race. The concept is not included into various religious beliefs yet Anne Besant met Helena Blavatsky a couple of times and came over to India. She even left her husband, children and family behind. Her charismatic personality has been a leading light across India so that she even became the President of the then Indian National Congress. Her peaceful demeanour was having the roots into her firm belief, 'There is no hurry, howsoever work may be important there will always be a dawn tomorrow and if this is not completed in this life, it can always be finished in the next life.' The Buddhist belief has the living symbol of the Dalai Lama. He is having his 14th birth now and as long as the people of Tibet will need a protector, he has vowed himself to be born again and again.

For most Indian people rebirth is as evident as the palm of their hand. A living example is Dr. Dipankar Patra, Vice President of the Indian Society for Clinical and Experimental Hypnosis. When his adolescent boy was not steadily successful in his collegiate career, he found out with age regression to the past life that his sensibilities rested in fine arts and film making. So he even shifted the young man to Mumbai where apart from being successful, he is living an enjoyable life.

For a hypnotherapist, thus past life regression is a last resort where metaphors have not succeeded. Thus, this is one of the final tools that may be used as a strategy to reorient a dysfunctional person. We usually answer the patients asking, 'do you believe in rebirth?' by saying 'If you believe that the life after life is a continuous process and your *Karmic* connections of past life have profound relevance to present life activity then we are agreeable to try the last strategy out to help you to live a useful, productive life.'

Session 2 (Anu)

(Client's detailed history is taken and noted year and if need be, monthwise, to give suggestion. Later on it may be ascertained that she did experience.)

The history taking goes this way in detail suggestions can be formed:

History as told by subject in awake state:

Born - Aug 3rd 1975

2007 March - Joined Hypnotherapy course.

Jan - Went to Allahabad to attend *Ardh-kumbh* meet Pavani and met Shri Rameshbhai Oza and Swami Chidanand Saraswati.

2006 Dec - Went to Mysore and Ooti.

Nov - Went to Varanasi and visited Laheri Baba's house.

July - Served Daynand Saraswati and attended lectures on Vedanta.

June - Joined SVYASA.

March - Finished course of Kaivalya Dhama.(University)

2005 Nov - Went to Ranchi.

July - Joined D.YED at Kaivalya Dhama.

May - Went to Ranchi for 1 month, had a very good experience in Meditation. Swami convinced me to continue with my studies or join some course.

April - Came back home from Rishikesh with the entire luggage.

1999 Dec - Read biography of Yogi for the first time.

Oct - Read *Ramcharitra Manas*

1998 May - Left home for Rishikesh.

March - Started listening some *shlokas* in dream. Started having some strong intuitions regarding things which happened.

1997 - Started Thakur seva.

1996 - Went to Varanasi without informing family. Finished graduation in Fashion Designing.

1995 - Decided not to get married, in search of a *Guru*. Realized that I HAVE SOME DIFFERENT MEANING TO EXISTENCE.

1994 - Finished 12 and brother got married.

1993 - Started reading Osho.

1992 - Completed 10th and sister got married.

1991 - Changed the school.

1990 - Started liking spiritual scriptures and books.

1988 - Went to Singapore.

1985 - Visited Vrindavan for the first time with all family members and remembered everything that I saw when again I went back.

The subject is put into trance by quick induction technique and the trance was then deepened.(refer to deepening techniques.)

The subject is asked to hold the pen in the right hand. She is asked to sign at each particular junction of life. Later on this is compared with the subject as to how at that age S signed and is confirmed when S is fully awake. From the time that child has held the pen to the time of induction of trance.

As is evident, the signature changes with age and also the language like from vernacular to the present state may be English or otherwise.

Anu, kindly keeps watching yourself and when it is alright, and when it is alright for me to take over; you may please give me your kind consent by signing your name. Very, very nice and since you have consented, shall we now carry on our work, a further forward, (C T) or sometimes further is back and back is sideways. But as we make this random movement, I want to know, are you prepared to go back in time when you were at a place in Taragini hall (previous day session)? May be, it was evening before yesterday. (DT). Then and then only, when you are wanting to say, 'yes', Please hold the pen with your hand and then when you are in Targini hall, day before yesterday, now she is in T hall and she has fresh memories of having performed the *pooja*, meditation in meditation centre contemplation and as you watch the train passing several such stations, as Feb 07, at the station at a glimpse Jan 07, yes, it is a fast moving train there is Allahabad. There is Kumbhmela that is going on. You see Shri Rameshbhai (a Hindu scholar) face to face 'such a gifted, wonderful, pleasant person.' She is a very spiritual person that she signs her name. When Rameshbhai is there, you also see brilliant, luminous face of *Chidanand* (Ecstasy) and receive his blessings too.

Your train is moving fast and we want to go miles and miles at a faster pace, much, much at a faster speed, such that as you reach at a faster speed, you are in July 2006. You are in the spiritual presence of Dayanand Saraswati at Prashanti Kutiram (name of the place). You sign in his presence. This place has been familiar and we were here only 2 days back (CT).

Anu has a choice when Anu wants to go slow and it's your choice to go slow. Anu will move any of her fingers of right hand if she wants to go slow. But Anu wants to move fast, she is in Nov 2005, she is in Ranchi. Anu gives consent to move fast and she is already in Ranchi. She sees herself in Ranchi, in Nov 2005. It's a beautiful place. There are various *Ashrams*, and temples. She meets many saints, sages, *gurus*, and learned people. They are radiant spirituality all around you now and this spirituality is getting richer and richer and further rich by presence of Anu. She feels fine fragrance surrounding her all around. When it is May 2005, we are in Ranchi and you are experiencing aesthetically spiritual experience in meditation. When you feel that spiritual fragrance and, as you are feeling that spiritual fragrance, Anu certifies that by her signature that, Anu is feeling that fragrance.

Please Anu, as you have done such an intense work in such a short time, you are being helped to sign. Please hold the pen and sign it. Now please stay at Ranchi. It is a serene, quiet, peaceful, tranquil place. Please meditate here all by your self. In that meditation there is silence and stay in that silence for a while till we decide to go to Rishikesh.

Stay in the state of meditation, you are not hearing my voice any more nor you hear any other sounds around you. There is only a sound of fine fragrance, a sound of subtle fine fragrance. My voice has gone further and further far away.

Anu is in deep trance so other participant is asked to ask any question. Even if they do not have, they ask to confirm later on that she has not listened the dialogue.

(During the session, participants are encouraged to ask questions and discussion occurs. Later on, after waking up the subject, it is confirmed that she was so deep in trance that she did not hear anything spoken by the participants.)

Q. She is not listening to our voice. How will you take her out of Hypnosis?

A. You will see it shortly.

Q. Why do you do Age regression and how do you prepare the subject?

A. We get the full history and also there is a dialogue, consent and full information is gathered. The subject writes down in detail with dates the important incidences of life. They will be happy or sad events (like death of near and dear one or major accidents) which are relevant. The events are written in reverse manner, e.g. she writes from 2007 march. Usually, the subject says that he or she neither does nor remember the event. At that time she needs to be encouraged as it may be in deep unconscious as repressed event.

"When the symptom started; Say 1995, does not remember. We have to age regress till 1993 when she was completely well. Asking; something happened in 96, 97 when Anu was connected with it. (Giving her a gentle touch on forearm sometime helps to recollect. A gentle touch assures the subject that therapist is walking with her.)

(EG) Once you are with the therapist (Name of the therapist) once again, you are in such a wonderful state of meditation; this is the gift of being Spiritual person. We may go to RISHIKESH.

If you want to go please indicate (ID). If you wish to go please sign your consent. Take your own time. (The subject is in deep trance and is taking longer time. Please be patient. Even ask her to move left finger if she does not wish.) She is taking longer time. So the therapist with the firm tone says; I am asking Anu, simple question that either go to Rishikesh or think that we had enough of work. Stay where you are and you are not listening to me.

As she is not answering, she is in very deep trance, the therapist can take own decision. The goal is to go to past life.

The therapist once again talks to the subject. (EG) Anu, it is nice, radiant spiritual glow on your face. Your face is shining with that glow. We have set a goal of going to past birth. And when you are ready, please sign your consent. She signs. Thank you so very much.

You want to go to past life, further and further, to go far far away. Now that you have started going, it is fast approaching and is about to approach. We go fast and faster and may be several years backward. We decide to go with the speed of light (3), and than little slower than the speed of light, you see many *Ashrams*, and you see that you have visited a few of them. You have been there and you are witnessing it. You have put up for few days at Devprayag and few days at Badrikedar (north India). You are moving fast and you are at Baroda (West India) and still faster you are at Rameshwar (South India) and Chitrakut. Here, how nice it is to witness *Krishna Leela*.

You are at Nasik (These are all holy places of India). But you are so spiritual that you are at the holy river Ganga at Rishikesh. You are at the holiest of all the holy places, where all Hindus (depending on faith, Vatican for Christian, Mecca for Muslims etc.) would wish to stay. All the Hindus and such other people who believe in spirituality, her heart is filled with joy at Varanasi. You are vast event of Mahakumbh Mela. Having had all this spiritual enunciation with all these holy man, you are going at a high speed and a faster rate. It is year 1996; she is a naughty girl of 22 years. She decided not to get married. She went to Vrindavan without informing parents. They were worried as to where she has disappeared. But that was to be as family does not know what the aim of Anu is. She is a different person.

It is year 1994. Anu is very happy for 2 reasons. Brother is married. She finished her 12th std. It is just a simple jump of proton particle. Proton particle has no mass. It also jumps like waves also. She knows all the stuff like electron. It is 10th std. She passed her 10th std. The other event in life and it is year of sister's marriage. You have a choice now. Either you are in Singapore in a school trip or at Vrindavan. As you have made a choice, you need not tell me your choice.

May be it is year 1998, or may be 1995, or 1990 or 1985, whatever is your choice, Anu holds the pen and signs her name and certifies once again.

Now, Anu, I am so happy to work with you. I have a great privilege to be associated with you. With one quantum jump of the proton particle Anu is going to Aug. 3rd 1975 (Birthday).

The, The, The very day, yes, such wonderful day, Aug. 3rd 1975, and now Anu is travelling at speed of light, in a wink of an eye, Anu sees herself in her mummy's tummy. It is July 1975, June, April, and March, so comfortable in mummy's tummy. The tiny Anu, a tiny dot (3), a little beautiful tiny dot in December 1974, and now Anu goes with the speed of proton or even faster than proton. It is 1974 Nov. 1973, 1972, 1971, 1970, 1969, 1965, 1960 and as far beyond, as far as you like to go. May be at 10 MB, 20 MB may be 15 MB (CONFUSION), and little less than 100 years, India is in turmoil, 1856, the war of independence. It is whole of North India, West India, it is here and there.

Anu is more or less there. She sees what she wants to see, what is she, then and now. In 1986 like speed of light you dart forward 130 years forward and backward and it is 1855 and please write what you want to write.

Yes you are my friend. We are great friends but I have forgotten your name. "Will you please write your name". She is under deep trance. She is regressed to past birth. But still she signs her name as of today. My dear friend, you are a spiritual person and has great spiritual aspiration. You want several phases of past birth, evidently face to face to yourself. (At these stages you have to avoid transference and counter-transference by saying "it is your doing, I am just walking along you etc.)".

You are going so fast. I find it rather difficult to travel with you. So I stay behind (ejecting the subject to be independent). You go for further journey, 200 years, 500 years, and 1000 years or years of astronomical figures. All these you are seeing are like a flash of light. This was your prerogative. This is your natural due. It is a special privilege for Dr. Rajni and Dr. Bhaskar Vyas to have accompanied you so far, and far beyond.

But we have promises to keep and we make the promise that the memory of this sublime spiritual experience will remain fresh and alive with you, whenever and that every time you want or wish to experience, you will be able to do so in a jiffy.

Let us turn back, fast, faster with a speed of light now from wherever we are in time, space and consciousness, your consciousness is returning back. Now you are returning back to the place where you started (Ashwini hall) at NIMHANS.

You are wonderful, great, and supremely spiritual with such a sublime experience now you are pristine pure. Now you will listen to Rajni.

Anu, now gradually you are waking up, but all that you have experienced is yours to keep. My voice (Dr. Vyas) is going silent. Though I am still sharing spiritual experience with you. We had a long journey back and so we are turning back to the Ashwini hall with a speed of light. Yes you are fully relaxed, peaceful, comfortable.

As I count from 5 to 1, you open your eyes, awake, fully awake, all that you have experienced is stored with in you, in your mind, in your brain. I count 5—4—3 and as I am counting backward, take your time to walk in to Ashwini hall, wide awake, alert and fresh in yourself and having all the fragrance that you had during the journey. 3—2—, yes Anu, you are feeling light in your eyes, you try and work to open it, and they want to open it, allow it to open. Wide awake, and on count of 1, 2—1, and Anu Open your eyes (command). Open your eyes and start breathing normally. Try and move yourself. Alert and wide awake.

She then travelled by bus and she was in trance state for 3 days. Attendant was by her side for her daily needs. She worked in that meditative phase and when she reported back after 3 days, she declared that she has made her decision and she will go to Vrindavan and live there as *Braj Gopi*. She was fine and happy. After two months, she was happy to have taken the decision.

Age regression

For several mental disorders, diseases and syndromes, the diagnosis is often unclear. Psychiatrists debated Diagnostic and Statistical Manual for Mental Disorders (DSM) classification for several years and in 2013 a 5th edition was published. In 2022, a further text revision was published by the American Psychiatric Association.

American Psychiatric Association was ahead of British Psychiatric Association to recognize hypnotherapy as one of the ways psychotherapy can help mental maladies.

DSM is intended for psychiatrists so that they can diagnose mental disorders and formulate case assessments that lead to an informed treatment plan for each individual. The case formulation for any given individual should involve a careful clinical history and concise summary of the social, psychological, and biological factors that may have contributed to developing a given mental disorder.

While the psychiatrists have toiled several decades to arrive at DSM 5, still uniformity in diagnosis evades this discipline with a litmus test. It is not unusual for two psychiatrists to disagree with each other about the diagnosis. On the other hand, more and more newer molecules have been discovered in the New Age. What was thought as a contraindication, such as severe depressive state and schizophrenia, they are also now being treated with drugs and supportive psychotherapy such as hypnotherapy.

While establishing the diagnosis and initiating its treatment with drugs is left to the psychiatrist, hypnotherapy is found to be highly supportive. Thereafter patients not only live a useful, productive life but can have children in a marriage.

We have devised a model applicable to most mental disorders. The model was presented at Bremen, Germany in 2013 and thereafter has been practiced by us and others. The steps involve a few well established phenomena as: 1. Quick induction with high rapport, 2. Deepening of the trance, 3. Age regression to the time when the first symptoms of the malady were noticed, 4. Re-living of any distressful situations at that time, 5. Catharsis for sufficient time, 6. Selective ablation of the traumatic event, 7. Substitution with a pleasant, enjoyable event before the trauma, 8. Age progression only with pleasant memories to the present, 9. Progression into the future with enjoyable, pleasant daily life with productive activities.

The strategy for the age regression is described below:

> History of the patient: 22 years old subject was suffering from migraine since 2015 (5 years). He was a psychology student pursuing sports psychology, was exposed for the first time to hypnotherapy in a workshop. So he was motivated to be relieved from the migraine through hypnotherapy. The subject was put into trance and the precipitating cause was not explored and age regression was done after knowing the year of onset.

(Induction by PMR, Deep breathing.)

Yes. Take a deep breath... deep breath... and as you take a deep breath and relax... deeper and deeper breath still and as you are relaxing now, the weight in your right hand starts diminishing. Your right hand is getting lighter and lighter and lighter. It wants to float... float... Without my support it is dropping into your lap... Niraj... very nice... thanks for the trust... thanks for the confidence and thanks for the friendship. Now that you are in a rapid mode, now that you are in a rapid mode, the muscles in your neck are totally relaxed and both the eyes have eyelids. These eyelids are now so tightly closed... Niraj has 2 eyes with 2 eyelids and they are tightly closed so Niraj is finding it difficult to open his eyes. Niraj, try to open your eyes and find that your eyelids... your eyelids are heavier... getting even more heavy and heavier that as if they were lead curtains. As if they were lead curtains. And now that we have begun the work in a rapid action mode, we are in a rapid action mode and Niraj has a choice to let me know whether he is Niraj is surely wanting to get a cure for his migraine. If really so, Niraj, let me know by moving any of the fingers of your right hand. Your choice and I surely will honour your choice that you want which is your natural due and if there is the natural due, it will surely accrue. Accrue to Niraj today and now. You see yourself Niraj, seated in a easy chair at Parimal building on a second storey and as you know, you have a 3rd eye and I am now opening your 3rd eye at your Agnachakra between 2 eyebrows. Niraj is seeing himself seated in a easy chair at Parimal. When Niraj sees himself as getting up from this chair, Niraj has gotten up from this chair, proceeded towards the staircase. Proceeded towards the staircase and Niraj is wondering. Oh there are two staircases and there are steps that I want to climb down. Niraj wants to climb down the staircase and from the step 2020, there is a step marked as 2020 and Niraj is climbing down 1 step to 2019. 2019 December... November... October... It has been so much full of wonder to live in Vadodara learning, studying at MS University and June 2019... April 2019... and Niraj takes 1 step further down with his 3rd eye now in a rapid action mode. There may be rapid action but at an important event... at an event that is important in 2018 and it has been really troublesome to keep on having this migraine attacks every now and then. One side of Niraj's head really starts getting so painful and it has been painful now and another step down backwards to 2017. See one side of your head getting painful. What a bother! What difficulty! It is really troublesome.

One more step down and 2016. Yes, yes, real trouble, real headache. And Niraj wants a rapid action and he gets further down 2 more steps... 2015... 2014... 2013... and the migraine is clearly evident. There is a one side of the head is aching, bothering, not allowing Niraj to work and he cries out, "Oh God, why are you so bothersome to me?" And even when Niraj cries for help to whatever God that may be, God does not answer and Niraj feels like going down in a rapid action mode further few steps. 2013... 2012... 2011... 2010... and the headache is really intense. The half side of the head is hurting so very hard that Niraj cries out to the father in heaven and to his father on earth. "Oh God, oh father, why hast thou forsaken me? Why hast thou forsaken me?" The headache is intense, the pain is real grief and the grief is touching the heart of the heart. The heart of the head at each and every cell in Niraj's body. "Oh father in heaven, oh father on the earth, why hast thou forsaken me?" And Niraj is hearing there is someone speaking from the sky. The god is answering Niraj from the sky, "I have never forsaken Niraj". You are seeing Christ, Niraj and you are the Christ. You are the Christ who carries his own cross on his shoulders and everyone has to carry his own cross on the side. And those who have carried the cross will be crucified on the very cross and then will resurrect." But Niraj as you are pondering, standing on the staircase, is it 2011... 2010... 2009... 2008... 2006... 2007... 2009... 2007... 2005. There is once again answer from the heaven. The God that is there in the heaven has never forsaken Niraj. Niraj is an eternal child and everybody who carries the cross. Everybody who has carried his own cross will certainly be resurrecting. Everybody who carried the cross... look at your own cross and be sure... as you look at your own cross, be sure that you will be resurrected. That moment, that moment that you identified your own disbelief and cried to the Father in heaven, "Why hast thou forsaken me?" Niraj forget, delete, eliminate this disbelief and when you have certainly forgotten this disbelief, move any of the fingers of the right hand. And when you are so sure that your disbelief is totally deleted, you have forgotten it altogether, you are not even able to move any of the fingers of the right hand. Good. Very good. I am really proud of Niraj that he can do so much of work in such a short time that he will now come back climbing rapidly some 15, 14 or 12 steps of Parimal's staircase and Niraj is rapidly climbing up the staircase steps so that he is on 2012... 2014... 2017... 2018 and he is in 2020 when he has so splendidly assisted in conducting and advance hypnotherapy workshop where he is convinced of the capabilities of hypnotherapy as a science and Niraj's future prospects to be one of India's leading sport hypnotherapist. Sport is really sportsmanly. The sportsmen take every game in their stride and at times there may be 1,00,000 people in a stadium and at times sportsmen play the game that sportsman like Niraj have. Niraj has so candidly played so that the bright future 2020 Niraj is getting qualified as a hypnotherapist and he will further advance into sports hypnosis. With new ventures, be it cricket, be it tennis, be it kho kho, kabaddi kabaddi kabaddi... And Niraj is now, at his discretion, when Niraj is sure of his very bright prospects as a sports hypnotherapist in making, then Niraj will wake up.

(Terminate the trance)

Migraine

Migraine has already been discussed earlier. It may therefore suffice to enlarge our understanding that there is no single cause for migraine. The cause lies in an unresolved conflict between two hemispheres of the brain.

Roger Sperry, operated on patients' brains that at times included severance of the corpus callosum. This would apparently mean that now right and left hemispheres cannot communicate with each other.

When a patient is having a migraine that expresses as a headache on one side of the head that means there is lack of coherence between the two hemispheres. A subject copes with this situation by suppressing the unsolved data into his unconscious mind. As we have well understood unconscious mind is truly the demiurgic, dynamic mind when the pressure on an unresolved conflict builds up beyond the coping limit, it surfaces in the morning as one sided headache.

It may be almost impossible to identify what is the unresolved conflict but a resolution with a metaphor may correspond to the unconscious mind that there is a solution to every unresolved conflict just as a simple question like "Why fish should not be spelled as Ghoti?" Solved the migraine of an English teacher lady.

The subject was relieved of her migraine for good. She wrote back in a couple of weeks with her experience, as follows:

This was my first experience of hypnotherapy. It was aimed at treating my migraine, a disease I lived with for more than 25 years. I am a 47 year old woman, troubled with migraine since my college days. I was given a therapy session by Dr. Bhaskar Vyas and Dr. Rajni Vyas in a hypnotherapy class in the presence of four students on March 17, 2019.

I went for the session with an open mind, with an intention to surrender completely to the therapists, expecting a trance that would take me to a level of consciousness where my body and mind would simply let go. Though I was aware that in trance one doesn't necessarily lose consciousness, I still had the idea that I would not be in control and my thoughts would be suspended under the influence of the therapist. But it was nothing that dramatic. In fact, I started doubting whether at all I was in trance, the reasons being the following:

1. A brief case history was taken which didn't seem adequate to me. I felt the therapist didn't know about me and my life sufficiently before starting with the induction.
2. I was given a very nice PMR that helped me to relax physically and to a great extent mentally as well. I can't say I was completely relaxed mentally because my thoughts or my logical brain was constantly at work. I was keenly aware of and distracted by the outside noise. Everything the therapist said, my mind, like Google, tried guessing beforehand. Any slips, deliberate or otherwise, were quickly detected by my active mind, though I desperately wished

that my thoughts would just shut up so that I could fully experience the peace I was being guided to.

3. There were questions that I had to answer. My mind frantically searched for the right experience in order to give the right answer. For example, I was asked to remember my favourite song sung by the legendary singer Manna Dey. I scanned my memory to come up with the right song to be played in my mind. There were quite a few that came up, but I was not satisfied as they were not exactly the ones closest to my heart. I was disappointed a little, with myself, as I had to make do with the ones that presented themselves to the surface of my mind. Then the character of Sarat Chandra Chattopadhyay's novel was also a letdown as I failed to picturize the strong female protagonist delineated there.
4. The sweet smell that I was suggested to experience did come to my nostrils, albeit only for a few seconds. As it vanished soon, I strove to retrieve it, but in vain. When I tried hard, I could only smell the food being cooked in the nearby kitchen. (Only later did I learn that for any out-of-the-world experience, one must not try, but allow it to happen naturally.)
5. When I was told to visualize a rainbow, I was at a loss. When the therapist described the colours of the VIBGYOR, he missed out green which my active mind immediately registered. And also the vibrant colours of the rainbow hurt my inner eyes that longed for a more soothing colour of the sky.
6. When I was told to feel that my hand was weightless and was going up against the gravity, my mind was amazed and watched in wonder that I was actually lifting my hand without consciously trying to do so. I felt happy thinking that the trance was actually settling in. Then I was told that my eyelids were heavy and I wouldn't be able to open it even if I tried. I had no intention to disprove the therapist, on

the contrary, in order to experience the wonder once more, I opened my eyes. I quickly shut them back, embarrassed to have opened the eyes in the middle of the session, hoping that the therapist hadn't noticed.

7. Halfway through the session, I suddenly broke out in a bout of cough. The therapist tried to ease my mind saying that it was good that I was coughing out the conflict within. My mind longed for a glass of water as I knew I was coughing because my throat was dry. It was a common thing that I experienced often in my sleep, a problem I had inherited from my mother. A drop of water always relieved it. I was thinking of all that in the process of coughing.
8. Later, after the session came to an end, I was led to a room inside to lie down and sleep off the trance. Lying there I was conscious of two things, one that I had a severe pain in my neck, two that the therapist was discussing my case with the students in the sitting room. As for the neck pain, I had developed it right at the beginning of the session due to a faulty sitting posture perhaps, and I realized that the pillows supporting my head were not evenly kept, when I came to lie down on the bed. There was a senior hypnotherapist sitting at my bed-side. She put me back into trance again for a few minutes. She gave me the suggestion for relief of the pain. When I awoke, I was relieved of the pain.
9. I kept lying with closed eyes. As soon as she left, I quickly removed the extra pillows. I waited for her to leave the room because I didn't want them to know that I was wide awake, contrary to their general feeling that I was lost in slumber. And also, I kept on listening intently to the discussion going on outside.

All of the above have been narrated to explain why I questioned myself whether I was at all in trance. Now I would like to share why I feel that in spite of my not experiencing any conflict within, that might have caused the ailment, or not having quietened the logical brain that kept on popping up with suggestions, reflections and analyses, I have been healed. I believed in the power of hypnosis, whether registered by the conscious mind or not. My belief was further strengthened when my neck pain was cured by Dr. Rajni Vyas within minutes by again applying the therapy in response to my complaint. Secondly, the positivity within me was greatly strengthened by the session. Finally, before going home, when I met Dr. Bhaskar Vyas, he very tenderly told me, 'Next Sunday if you come to me and report that you had no migraine, you win, I win. And if you get the headache, you win, I lose. Do you want me to lose?' Well, I had already accepted him as a father figure, and my father being very dear to me, I promised myself that I wouldn't let him lose the battle waged against my migraine. May be this is what is called Transference in psychotherapy. I did transfer my feelings towards my own father to the therapist. But I don't know if it was a by-product of the therapy. Elderly people remind me of my father and I develop a natural tenderness for them and respect them, even going so far as nurturing a protective feeling for them. I don't want them fail psychologically. So, I am not sure if the love and attachment I felt for my therapists were sown by the hypnotherapy session or my inbuilt tendency.

What transformation as a human being I had, I cannot tell, as, till date I have no inkling whether any hidden conflict, if there was any, was resolved on that day. But I take every opportunity to learn and grow, improving myself in the process. So, from that point of view, the session certainly was a learning experience that contributes to my being a better person in life. One thing I firmly believe, and that is, **I have been healed.**

My Return to Reality

I don't think I was diverted from reality even for a moment. I do realize that it is my own belief; my faith in healing that will keep me well in future. My therapists have shown me the way. I do imagine them on both sides, protecting me from another migraine attack, and I keep reminding myself of my resolve not to let them down. But these are my ways to strengthen my mind. This is I suppose the reason why people cling to religion or *gurus*—just to fortify themselves against their own weaknesses, when they tend to buckle under pains, diseases and other stressors of life.

History: Subject was highly intelligent, brilliant in her perception, came with history of migraine since 10 years. Between 2 sisters, she thought that she is not good looking—dark, which was a taboo in her mind. She was extremely sensitive and all the time looking for remarks which were not really addressed to her. She thought that the mother did not like her looks.

She came for the workshop and thought that somebody remarked about her. She broke down completely and left the hall. She was attended by senior hypnotherapist for almost 45 minutes to convince her to attend the workshop. Finally, she stayed back, had 4 sessions. Later on, was supported by other 2 sessions to take her forward in her career of post graduation in medical science. She is progressing very well in her career. Migraine never bothered her for last 3 years.

(Induction using PMR, deep breathing)

You have been such a clever student right from your high school levels all throughout now in medical. All the time you have scored high ranks. Now, somebody who is clever, and excellent in everything that she does, she has only a little assignment today and that is... that is... India is going to defeat Corona for sure. And after some time Corona will go away from India, and migraine will go away today for good from Barkha. That's a agreement between three concerned parties. One is Barkha, another is uncle Bhaskar Vyas and third is the migraine. Now Barkha has read something yesterday about the right side of the brain... Barkha, yes. You are having migraine on the left side of the body... left side of the forehead, and that time Barkha will put her finger. Right now Barkha is putting one of the finger... one of the finger of her left hand on the superficial temporal artery. Barkha knows where is superficial temporal artery? It is in front of the ear... When you know where is the tragus on the ear, just a little anterior to the tragus, Barkha is able to palpate her superficial temporal artery.

Yes Barkha, palpate your superficial temporal artery and see how nicely... in a regular rhythmic and without any kind of pain around that superficial temporal artery, it is pulsating. Yes, Barkha?

That's very nice. Now, we are going to give several commands. Keep your hand on the superficial temporal artery and keep on feeling the pulsation of the superficial temporal artery and with each beat of that artery... that artery is pulsating... the artery is pulsating so regularly... the artery pulsation is regular and all the volumes of pulses... each pulse of that artery, feel the volume of the pulse Barkha and verify for yourself that the pulsation... the pulsation of the arteries are all equal in volume. And as you find good pulsations, they synchronize with your breathing and take a deep breath... deep and even deep breath. Deep and even deep breath and... and with each deep breath, there are 4—1... 2... 3... 4 pulsation in the temporal artery. And as you take deeper and deeper breaths, the pulse rate is now going down. The pulse rate has gone down... deeper breaths and deeper breaths still then with each deep breath, now there are 1, 2, 3, 4, 5 pulsations in the artery. And what a marvellous demonstration that Barkha... Barkha not only can take a deep breath, Barkha is taking deeper and deeper breaths and as she has demonstrated to herself that she can slow down... slow down... sloowww down. Slow down the beating of her own heart. The heart rate has gone down and it is beating in a regular fashion... in a regular fashion with each pulsation in the same volume but the heart rate has gone down from 72 to 70 and from 70 to 68... 65... 64... 66... 67... 65... 62... and her eyes, Barkha's eyes have been really very very heavy. Very heavy eyelids and why... why do we have to struggle to keep them... keep them open? We don't have to struggle for anything and let your eyes close. Let your eyes close and again Barkha has closed both her eyes and how nice to relax... Re...

Lax... Relax... Relax... In the sole of both the feet.. Relax in both the feet. All the muscles in the feet, not only the extensor hallucis longus and extensor hallucis gravis has relaxed... but interossei the small muscles between each and every phalanx... see the interossei in the feet... in both your feet and feel them relaxing. Barkha has learnt a mastering control whereby she can relax not only the interossei in both the feet but with one deep breath, deeper breath still... Take a deep breath Barkha... And with this deep breath, feel the relaxation spreading in both your feet and both the legs. In both your thighs. Way up in your girdle. In front of the chest. In the back of the chest. And way up onto the cervical spine and right up to... right up to the superficial temporal artery on the left side where you had put your fingers. Let those fingers also relax... Re lax... Re... laxx. And let the superficial temporal artery also relax. So that. So that Barkha is now at total rest. Happy by herself... Happy for having been a medical student. Happy having been such an excellent person and happy in her own happiness. Barkha is happy in her own happiness and as happiness has spread all over the brain... Barkha's both the hemispheres of the brain... the right and the left and the left and the right are connected... are very firmly and soundly connected with a corpus callosum... and the brain structure is been seen. Barkha is now seeing both the hemispheres of her own brain... The right side of the brain is to talking to the left side and the left side is talking to the right side... Let let the dialogue between two sides of the brain prolong into a mutual convergence so that.. so that now... now Barkha is able... able to open... Barkha has two eyes. Both the eyes are closed. But between two eyes, Barkha has a third eye. Barkha... dear child... the most excellent... most excellent person... brilliant medical student has opened her third eye located somewhere between the two eyebrows and the third eye.. the third eye has a span... the right eye and the left eye can see near and far.. The third eye that Barkha has opened has a span that sees between 2020... and she sees 2020 March beginning... when she perceived a resurgence of migraine headache... migraine headache... once again came to Barkha and Barkha is having pain on the left side of the head right now... Barkha, the right side of your head and some of the part of the face and the jaws on the right side are having pain... But the right eye in a flash... in a flash has gone to January 2020... and what a beauty! What a mastering control... the Barkha has opened her third eye and she sees January 2020... Her migraine is gone.

The left side that was having headache and the pain has vanished with a look from the third eye... and Barkha your third eye is viewing all those situations... the situations in 2019... that gave you severe migrainous headache. With rapid pulsating string like contraction of superficial temporal artery, and all those situations are vividly passing in front of 3rd eye of Barkha. December 2019, November 2019, July 2019, March 2019, December 2018, and in rapid succession Barkha is viewing all those painful situations that gave her this situation. 2018, 2017, 16, 15, 14... yes and you can look backward and forward with the 3rd eye and see those situations once again with in 2016, 15, 14, 13, 12 and 10... here is Barkha, the lovely adolescent child on the verge of teenage and when she looks at 2019, that was really troublesome and 2009, lovely, innocent, chirpy, ebullient, happy with delight is Barkha. She is seeing... her 3rd eye is seeing a lovely, innocent child in 2009. There was no migraine. What was that migraine? With one sweep, one blink of your 3rd eye; Barkha blink both your eyes and let your 3rd eye also blink. And with that blink... Barkha's blink of her 3rd eye, everything that was unpleasant... everything that was causing a conflict, everything that could not be resolved, with that one blink all that caused the migraine; it is suddenly wiped off. Wipe off... wipe off... wipe off the memories of unresolved conflict. Wipe off the conflicts altogether. All conflicts unresolved have suddenly been wiped out of your memory and the memory of the innocent Barkha of 2009 now prevails and pervades so that the innocence spreads and Barkha is seeing the spreading of that innocence. That innocence has a fragrance. The fragrance of innocence. Take a deep breath and deeper breath still and feel a fine fragrance of innocence in both your nostrils. Take a deep, deep breath. Feel the fine fragrance of innocence spreading from 2009 to 2010, 12, 11, 14, 15,... what a clever rapid movement. Child is blossoming into adolescence and into a full blooded feminine form so that the innocence has now spread to January 2020 and that 2020 January prevails all the way up to April 2020. Keep on feeling that fine fragrance of innocence and as we go with your 3rd eye open to April and May 2020 and 2020 Barkha is a brilliant medical student. Blossoming out to be a prospective brilliant student and 2021, 2022 Barkha is shaping to be one of the best dermatologists that India would have ever produced. This is not only my promise to Barkha but Barkha's own tryst with her destiny. And such a tryst of destiny will have several colours. Several colours ranging from orange, red, yellow, to different kinds of blues, violet, navy blue but the most mystical black... the black colour with a shining glow is truly mystical and that mystery will unveil in whatever that Barkha will do from now on. My privilege. I am so happy. Rajni aunty and I are privileged to have confidence of Barkha and while Barkha is relaxing... Barkha is resting having done such wonderful work.

Confidence Building

You are so talented that you can do any of the subject that comes your way. That is my blessing. Do you believe that blessings come true?

Yes sir.

When the giver is fully empowered and the recipient is fully ready to receive. If the recipient has a doubt, then it won't happen. If they are sure it would happen then it will happen for sure. If there is going to be a dawn tomorrow, you don't say hope there will be a dawn tomorrow. Are you sure of the dawn tomorrow or are you hopeful of a dawn tomorrow?

I'm sure of dawn tomorrow.

So, you may not remember what we did this January with Barkha. But there is a special kind of empowerment; Rajni also worked with you and I also worked with you. So, this is the kind of special gift we gave to Barkha last January 2020. Now, I take it forward that this is kind of a sure and certain ability that Barkha has. Barkha has a sure and certain ability and this ability has a potency. Sometimes when Barkha takes a deep breath and lets it go as if she has put a nisasa. Nisasa is nihi asha. When she feels doubt about any situation that otherwise she would have been competent, absolutely sure and certain competent but sometimes she gets surrounded when negative thoughts. How will this happen? Will I be able to do this or not? Then this comes as gheraod. A word in Indian English. Barkha has known this and there is another aspect of Barkha that the moment there are a few feelings of raindrops, Barkha is a soothing rain. A cooling rain and Barkha certainly brings *bahar* with herself. So, when Barkha would once in a while as a medical doctor, as a medical student, she wouldn't like to put any *bindi* on her forehead. Barkha may not like to put a *bindi* on her forehead but Barkha has learnt she is already learnt and familiar with how she will enhance not only reveal but she will enhance her self-potential that is Barkha's natural due. It is natural due of Barkha to relax, relax, and even more relax. She takes a deep, and deeper still breath and she feels a confident relaxation all over her body. Perfect poise and with so much increase in oxygenation... deeper and deeper breath... Barkha has taken a deeper breath, the oxygen saturation has jumped up to 99%. 9... 9... is 99%. Oxygentaion gives so much vigour, vitality and clarity of mind. Now she wants this to be enhanced to a superlative brilliance. So, this is the gift that Rajni aunty and Bhaskar uncle and your mommy. Barkha as a medical student, as a doctor, is a high professional person and a professional etiquette is optional. Rajni aunty also and maybe your mommy as well, once in a while they have put a *teeka* or a *bindi* somewhere in the lower part of your forehead. Once in a while if you go to a party, you go to a marriage celebration and you have to dress up. You may as well are fully entitled to dress up with a *bindi* on your forehead. That is a natural attribute that must occur to every Indian lady. However, professionally there are situations. Take a deep, deep, deep breath. There are professional situations where you are challenged and you cannot dress up professionally to show off a *bindi*. In the situation, move the left index finger, that is the first finger in your left hand. And as you know what is the left hand, and you know what is the left index finger, move the index finger of your left hand. When the left index finger, the index finger of the left hand, touches the left thumb you are, *'ye kya ho raha hai?'(what is happening?) samaj main nahi aata,(Don't understand)* but my left index finger wants to touch my left thumb. For a moment your left index finger and the left thumb, they come into contact. They have come into a contact with each other. T-O-U-C-H—TOUCH and with the touch of index finger and the thumb, with the touch of index finger and the thumb, about 100 immediate early aroused genes; genes are the ultimate dictator. They dictate our behaviour. Genes dictate our behaviour and when thumb of the left hand has touched the left index finger of Barkha, they are not able to separate each other and at this very moment, there is a certain and sure appreciation as if there is a *tikka,* there is a *bindi* in Barkha's forehead. Feel the transference of empowerment. Em-power-ment... your real, confident, sure, certain self that radiates brilliance, certainty from your forehead to all over the brain and to your autonomic nervous system is empowered. Sympathetic system is cooled down and stay confident and stay sure and be certain that this gift, you may invoke any time and every time when you need brilliance, vigour, vitality, surety in your performance. Rajni aunty and Bhaskar uncle feel proud of Barkha. Such a highly intelligent and most successful doctor to be for sure.

All the best Barkha, stay relaxed, maybe go to sleep. Stay relaxed and stay confident.

Stress Relief

- **30 Y/o M.A Economist—1 Year diploma in Spain.**
- **Worked for 3 years in Delhi and few years in Bombay.**
- **Felt low esteemed by colleagues and mother and went into depression.**
- **Resigned the job and went back home.**
- **Suggestion: Throwing stress out and building confidence.**

Today you are looking very fresh Ankit and I am so happy to see a different Ankit who has combed his hair nicely and nicely 1 tuft is coming on his forehead. And Ankit has a big forehead where his frontal lobe is the seat for consciousness and your consciousness is expanding and expanding and feeling very very fresh. Ankit, I am so happy that you are a very very quick learner, very confident, appreciated by people who have worked with Ankit but Ankit is running very fast. So, he is slowing down to the medium speed and he will soon get the order from the person with whom he has worked or he will be making a new application because Ankit is unique and very very hardworking, intelligent, having very clear intellect. Yes, you know this word and in Sanksrit it is called 'Pragnya'. His Pragnya is awake, alert... awake, alert and he is seeing through this Pragnya which is part of what is called as third eye in Sanskrit. It is in the shining forehead of Ankit in front of his two eyebrows. It is called the third eye or 'Agna Chakra' or centre for Pragnya.

And when he is sitting in the position of meditation, he is a meditator and with the closed eyes, through his third eye, eye of 'Agnyachakra', he is visualizing the whole, the whole 'Aakash'. Yes, this is really a Yogi taking, absorbing the energy from Sun God. Sun is his favourite who always has been accompanying Ankit. Yes, if you feel the same way Ankit, that the Sun is moving with you and awakening your third eye which his centre for Pragnya. You have been working through Sun god, please indicate with your finger. (ID) Yes Ankit, very nice. Wonderful. You have an equipment in your right thumb and index finger. Your Sun god is available to you when the thumb and index finger meets. Let the thumb and index finger meet. Very nice. Very nice. It is with you every time and anytime. Every time and anytime it is with you. Feel comfortable. You can move yourself here and there. Yes, and you are convinced about your ability, efficiency in the work, about the knowledge of economics that you have inherent in yourself and you learnt in college. Got M.A. and then from the Western University and back to India, the motherland, where motherland India has so many fresh entrepreneurs where Ankit is valued so high. Yes Ankit. I am so proud of you because Ankit is proud of himself. Confident, efficient and a very hardworking Ankit. Ankit got confident and more confident when former boss asked him to join back. And Ankit is now very much convinced about his abilities, his efficiencies, his knowledge, his Pragnya which now he is appreciating and has been certified by his former boss. He has finished his CV. He has got 1 job offer and he will be answering back; but in the meantime Ankit is ready to make other applications as well. Whatever will be best suited, Ankit will gather up and join back to the job of his choice where he will stick to that job and rise up in the position, in the pay and feel very well settled as now he is sure of himself that he is a gifted child, a gifted child of Almighty where Sun God awakens his Pragnya all the time and every time that he is working. Yes, very very nice Ankit, I can see your third eye open which is gathering, which is gathering all the energy. All the confidence, all the work power through his 'Agna Chakra' which is lying at the level of his 'Agna Chakra' and entering into his brain and all his nervous plexuses and he is a young, energetic entrepreneur. Yes Ankit, your face is shining through the Sun and if Ankit feels the same way, he will indicate with his finger. (ID) Yes, very nice Ankit, You are so confident of yourself. The same that Ankit is showing that self-confidence. Imbibe in your whole brain, in your consciousness for a minute till my voice disappears.

Ankit your face is glowing, your cheeks are pink, your forehead is shining with the sunrays that are entering through your Agnyachakra into your nervous system, your circulatory system and all that confidence is circulating through every crevices of your brain. All the convolutions. And the energy through the blood is circulating all over your body which makes young Ankit energetic, tranquil, quiet at the same time. Alert and ready to work with the help of Pragnya. Yes, Ankit feel this energetic Ankit for a while till my voice disappears.

Ankit today you have an awakening in your consciousness and it is spreading all around you into the whole sky which is described as '*Pruthvi, Api, Vayu, Teja, Aakash*' (5 elements with which body is made. Earth, water, air, light, sky) And has spread all over. Today your bed is wonderfully clean, creaseless and Yogi Ankit is sitting in Yogic position. All energized, fresh, ready to work and enjoy Ankit, this new energized, fresh, tranquil Ankit. Mummy and I, Dr. Rajni Vyas are very, very thankful to you to take us in this journey with you where our intellect also is awakened through Ankit. I am really, really very, very happy. Enjoy this trance; the 4th state of consciousness. The 4th state of consciousness which is bright, illumined, tranquil, quiet self of Ankit. Stay in this *Turya* state, 4th state of consciousness till you feel comfortable, quiet confident self. And I thank you and wish you all the best that is due to you Ankit and I am really proud of you Ankit. Stay and my voice quietens down as you are in this *Turya* state, the 4th state of consciousness. Enjoy till you like and wake up fresh, energized, ready to start your day. Whatever that is there in your brain, put it into the computer and ready to join the job you like between two offers. Ankit Thank you very much.

He woke up after full conviction of his capability and joined the job in two weeks from 1st of the month.

Devendra—History

Session 1

Confidence Building
(Introduction)
(History taking and rapport building)
Induction –

Praying to Devtas for help— asking permission from Devendra PMR, Deep breathing/ego strengthening suggestions.

When you were declared born, you were monitored for your heart sound and breathing by the doctor and then it has been going on and on and today you have a chance in your relaxed mode, listen to your heart sounds. It is so rhythmical, so regular and it is working so nicely. Please listen to your heart sounds as you are breathing. In and out. Take a deep breath Dev. Let that fresh energized oxygenated air into the smallest unit of your respiratory system and how wonderfully heart and lungs both the lungs and heart are working together, in a constant continuous way. Non-stop all 24 hours all round the year and keep on exchanging, you wonder you've never experienced this nice working of both heart and lungs and the whole body and observe yourself continuously seven days in a week 30 days in a month 365 days in a year, it continuously works and it keeps you alive, well, intellectually working and resting in 24 hours.

You listen to my voice and at the same time you experience, as you will experience this for a moment with the closed eyes I will be quiet.

Very nice. Very nice, Dev. Experience this quiet, peaceful moment in your routine, working, running about in this morning, please relax and experience this freshness with the closed or open eyes, whichever you like. You have heard and experienced moment experienced this rhythmic moment of your lungs and heart. If you have enjoyed this moment of life, please indicate. Very nice.

This relaxation wave moves on both the shoulders, both the hands and fingers and you can move your fingers throw out all your tension and all your worries. Let the sunlight bring the fresh energy to continue this relaxation wave to move from the neck high up into your face and neck. This neck connects, take a deep breath in and out, and it passes this fresh air into the small muscles of the face which relaxes and makes you feel younger by five years.

Your face relaxes your small muscle relaxes and it goes into the brain which is like a walnut with crevasses and it goes, this fresh oxygenated blood goes into the brain, the cerebrum the cerebellum, all the voices are going far away from you except my voice and you relax.

Take a deep breath in and out, in and out, and enjoy (2) this moment of relaxation. Wonderful. Very nice.

Dev you are a highly intelligent person, very creative, always working very hard for the humanity, the branch that you have chosen is what India needs today. The education for the young adolescent and adult this shows your personality of creativity and absolutely wonderful selfless activity which brings about great change in this that chaotic world that is existing at the moment all over, not only in India, but all over the world.

All that itching will go away and you are listening to my voice, I have great praise for your educational activities that I heard about you. Please relax and enjoy this state, my voice also quietens for a couple of minutes. Please enjoy this moment of relaxation.

Dev, I join you back in the journey of wonderful connection with the nature and this relaxation and yes, all that itch it's showing your ability to work for the social causes that you have imbibed from your parents as well as your education and you value this education from the experience of your life at a very, very young age.

Very, very young age in which you have shown your creativity, yes Dev, and if you like you can see your creativity with open eyes or closed eyes. For a while till my voice quietens.

Yes Dev, I am back with you and would you like to continue relaxing or would you like to wake up?

Dev, I have been with you and I would like to see your relaxed face, so Rajni has done so much of work with you which would have taken that much of work in a hardcore technological way would have taken 'X' Joules of energy that you have done in a few minutes, so I would like to reward you. Would you like to have some more rewards? So you have been in Bangalore and Bangalore is a city of gardens, would you like to go to Bangalore while sitting here wherever you are now? And with your closed eyes in a moment and in a jiffy, you can take yourself to your favourite garden in Bangalore.

Deeper, and deeper breath still. So in a jiffy, Dev has gone to a garden, his favourite garden, Lal Baug or whatever garden that Dev used to visit. Dev is now seeing what a blossom it is. What a blossom it is! The garden is full of various scents of flowers, these flowers are emitting a sweet perfume, a sweet perfume, that Dev is so very fond of. This sweet perfume gets stuck to your neck at the nape of your neck at the back, whole day today, whenever you scratch the nape of your neck, this perfume, the sweet favourite perfume for Dev, will permeate all around him.

Feel, feel the sweet perfume permeating through the mucosa of your nose. The permeating perfume of your favourite choice and you feel so relaxed, so relaxed. Dev has seen Violet flowers, Dev is seen indigo flowers, some of them are blue, some of them are green, some of them are brilliant yellow, they are so much yellow like the yellow sunflowers of Van Gogh. You have seen Van Gogh's painting of the sunflowers and you are seeing the same kind of sunflowers yes scratch your neck and as you're scratching your neck you are feeling the fine perfume of your choice permeating all around you. So as we were watching the yellow coloured sunflowers painted by Van Gogh. You have now closed your eyes, you are again scratching at the root of your nose and you are putting your favourite perfume there also. Every time during the day, you will scratch at the root of the nose, you will feel the same fine perfume of your favourite choice. Having worked so hard, I want Dev to relax by himself.

Yes this kind of intense work does make a person tired, but Dev is so wonderful a person, I will take up the matter whenever it is convenient for you to have a second experience whereby in this favourite garden of your choice we will take you in a split second, some 30 years back, hard to believe! Who would have thought that there would be jets and there would be supersonic jets. And so Dev is capable with his brilliant brain to work across, go over in time 30 years in a few seconds and delete all that was unpleasant. Dev, like pressing of the delete switch on the computer has deleted all that was unpleasant and he is once again back in the presence of the sacred band that he has on his right wrist that is for worshipping AGNI. We began with let the sacred fire of AGNI burn away whatever unpleasant, whatever unpleasant memory Dev may have some 30 plus years ago. For Rajni and Bhaskar Vyas this has been a great privilege to have worked with this young man with brilliant future. His future is being lit up by AGNI even this moment. Look at the glow on his face and his face is glowing like a brilliant red.

Yes, yes, thank you. Thank you Dev, for this the village and I will like Dev to have the pleasant memories of this experience and we look forward to work with you so as you eliminate whatever present stress of this mental situation you are harbouring.

Wake up now and let Dr. Rajni talk to you. Yes Dev you have been a wonderful person and should we help you to wake up completely and as I will start counting from 10-1, if you like you can keep your eyes open or if you like you can keep them closed. As I come to 1 as I come to 1, I'm counting from 10, 9... 8... 7 as I'm counting you are waking up from this trance state, your waking up, becoming alert and six... And five... Yes you are slowly waking up... And four... 3... 2 you are now alert, coming back to the present... And one.

Stretch yourself, move your head from side to side, yes Dev. Become alert, move your head from side to side, wonderful, forward and backward. Very nice. Stretch your hands, stretch your hands, both the hands. Now move your whole body sitting on the chair from side to side. Very nice. Having worked so hard, I want Dev to relax by himself.

Whenever you feel that you are likely to lose your temper, scratch the back of your neck and feel the fine perfume appear in your nose and your anger will disappear. As you scratch your neck and feel that perfume and your anger will disappear and the perfume will pervade. We will further so enhance that you will not get angry and we will further ensure that you go as a highly successful executive. That is our promise.

Thank you for listening patiently.

Session 2

(Ego strengthening—Guru Purnima) Anger control—Relation of Akhileshji

Dev, I'm so happy to see you so well and well composed and this auspicious day of Guru Purnima, we pay homage to all those *gurus* who have taught us this sublime and spiritual method of healing only with the words and we will want to take Devendra also on the same path that after some time they will gradually reduce the drugs, the dosage and eventually he will no more need any more drugs. Would you like to do that Devendra?

Now tell me Devendra, did you listen to the last session? So you have listened to the previous recording three times. Now Devendra, show me your right wrist and show me if you have done Agni *pooja* this morning, the red band is still there? Very good.

So they went through, you are really a privileged person. Devendra riding on a chariot, you are riding on a chariot. And the chariot, instead of being monitored with one *Sarathi* come on now Devendra you are showing me your right wrist and show me that there is red band which shows that you have performed the *pooja* as usual. You have tied the red band which is your protection band and I call it our *Agni Rath*. Now Devendra is all the time looking at the band on his right wrist and so is Ankita with eyes open. Ankita and Devendra are listening to Bhaskar Vyas, your friend philosopher and guide who is going to be making this couple who have married each other and devoted themselves with full devotion before this AGNI, the sacred fire,

ॐ भुर भुवः सव्ः। तत् सवितुरवरेण्यं।
भरगो देवस्य धीमहि। धीयो योनः परचोदयात्।।

And Ankita and Devendra as you listen to my chanting of this primordial *mantra*, the first to happen in this whole *Brahman*. *Brahman* is the entire cosmos, cosmos that has not only the earth and Jupiter and Venus and Mars and Uranus these are the planets. Planets are really small but the cosmos is so vast. With your eyes wide open, wide open... Yesterday NASA released a picture of the cosmos that had several stars and multiple stars including galaxies. What a *nazara*! (Wonderful panorama) Another is a special kind of viewing, we happen to see that kind of happening and when you see the whole cosmos now before your eyes, your eyes are saturated with satiety. Your tongue has passed on this satiety to your eyes and passed on the satiety to your tongue and so your eyelids have become so heavy, so very heavy, your eyelids I really heavy period...

It is difficult to hold them as open and if the eyelids are so heavy that they want to close, your eyelids are wanting to close. Feel even more relaxed.

Relax... Relax... Relax... Devendra, put your right hand on to the nape of the neck and as you put your right hand, you have put your right hand onto the nape of the neck. The same favourite kind of fragrance... The same favourite fine fragrance of Devendra's choice it's appearing in your nostrils and take a deep... Deep... And deeper still deep breath and the fine fragrance is pervading with every beat of your heart. Every beat of your heart throws fresh oxygenated blood along your body, along with this rejuvenating oxygenated blood, you are permeating each and every cell of your body with rejuvenating fragrance. You can change your position if you would, and become more comfortable resting your head back.

You can put your specs away because you will be seeing with your third eye. That is very nice. Make yourself comfortable. And as you take a deep, deep breath in, take a deep... Deep... Deeper still... Deep breath in. What a wonderful, definitely sublime blessing this is that your third eye has so opened that your other two eyes, their eyelids have decided to tightly shut. Both your eyelids have drooped down and your third eye opens and before the third eye there is Devendra in *pooja* clothes and Ankita sitting by his side are pouring with a large spoon, the sacred homage, homage that will be consumed by the fire, the fire is blazing bright now. You are seeing that the fire has lighted up and has blazing, blazing higher and higher up, consuming the offerings offered by Devendra and Ankita with folded hands. Ankita fold your hands, to bow down to pay *namaskar*, to pay *namaskar* to the sacred fire that consumes whatever that is offered to it with hearts open.

Devendra, the fire guard that is Agni, and Agni is consuming whatever with devotion, dedication and full faith Ankita and Devendra has offered to the fire. Fire is being lighted up and as the light of the fire goes brighter, you see around the fire someone like a monkey face. What is this monkey doing around here?

Devendra and Ankita are wondering and as Devendra is looking towards Ankita, and greater signs to Devendra that this is the protector deity that Ankita's father had requested to be present. We are hearing now a faint chant of Hanuman *stuti*, listen to the faint chant of Hanuman *stuti*. Both of you with folded hands pray to the protector deity, yes, both of you with folded hands pray to Hanumanji towards your highly purified mind and soul. Your mind and soul are so purified that anything bad, anything negative, anything that is likely to harm you has been taken away by Lord Hanuman and the fire will keep on blowing all the time and whenever Devendra is likely to experience any kind of bad thoughts, negative thoughts. You are a beautified person, you are now a spiritual, highly devoted person. A very well qualified engineer, and as you will scratch with your right hand that carries the fire band and scratch the nape of the neck. Devendra scratched the nape of your neck and a fine perfume pervades your body all over. Now, you are fully capable of providing, helping, providing sustenance to Ankita to Devendra and three of your very loved ones. One dog, and two newly arrived two daughters. So, Devendra is now providing, finding enough finances... Finance is money and money is the source of survival and sustenance. Every day Ankita has to spend for the family, for the food shelter and clothing and she has to save for the future of 2 young daughters, newly arrived in the family. Devendra is now finding sustainable employment whereby he is giving month by month money in Ankita's hand. Thus having evaporated anger, extinguished, consumed by the fire, now Devendra is fully equipped to go further with doctor Rajni Vyas. We are really privileged that we have this opportunity to work with such a wonderful couple who has given this chance for their redemption.

We move forward in the trance state and as you are listening to my voice with the 3rd eye, you are listening to my voice which is well connected with the brain, the hypothalamus and the pituitary. As it is whole, the third eye, the other name is *Agna Chakra* and it is at the same level of lower part of both the hemispheres

Hypothalamus, thalamus and pituitary, this anatomy you have heard many years back but these are the centres which control the whole body including the mind. As such mind has no place in the brain but each and every cell has a mind and it works in such a wonderful synchronous way and people like you who are so highly intelligent working very well and collecting the knowledge with the help of each other. But converting this knowledge into intelligence and being Indian... you can change your position, rest your back, put a pillow behind your head so that you are in a comfortable position... just relax and as you are making yourself comfortable and as you are touching your pet, ask the pet to be quiet, comfortable and touching you. You feel more and more comfortable, more relaxed, able to hear with your closed eyes and you are with yourself. And this intelligence is getting converted into wisdom. You are so intelligent, capable, able to collect all the information to convert into wisdom and that is how you are making the programmes of education which has been accepted for the teacher. You are highly intelligent and want to share your intelligence to the young generation who all are very very grateful to you and want to know more and more from your wisdom. You are Devendra, ahead of your time and the language that you use at times may be difficult for the listeners but for you it is so simple. Yes... because as I said you are ahead of your time. You will be patient, you will be compassionate and will explain little bit more at length to the people who are little less intelligent, less comprehensive and so you will have compassion and you will explain them patiently. In the process, some time you can become a little impatient and might get a little stressed out and anxious as to such a simple thing which is for Devendra is not being understood by your students. Devendra will have compassion. He will join his thumb and index finger and will be patient with all of them. There is a nice, pleasant chime hanging behind the computer where Devendra is sitting and the fine breeze comes which starts the syllable *Om* from the chimes. Yes, itch it out, throw it out. Getting more patient. Listening to this 'Om' chant and Devendra takes a little pause. The anger, the restlessness goes far, far away and Devendra is becoming cool, quiet within the self and starts explaining what he is conveying. At other times, he is watching a river which is flowing on both the banks in month of October. In month of October, after the heavy rains, the water is flowing smoothly, steadily with clean water and this flowing water makes Devendra very, very cool, comfortable. Watching the clear water where fish are flowing and as he watches these fish, he feels cool, comfortable and quiet within and feels very, very restful. He is teaching is flowing like this river and students are amazed to learn with the simple language of Devendra and Devendra feels very, very happy, cool, comfortable and joyful, tranquil and experience this joyful moment when my voice quietens down for couple of minutes. And my voice comes back and Devendra is enjoying this peaceful, quiet, tranquil moment when he listens to the morning *aarti* in the temple nearby and for good. Yes, you feel very, very quiet, comfortable. This soothing sound of *aarti.* Devendra fills up in his brain and passes it over to all the cells of the body and is ready to do his morning work from home of making the programmes for the students who value it very much because it is different from the other teachers, the other *gurus*, as it is full of wisdom that has been acquired by Devendra. He is all set with his computer, he is alert and he is composing in his self the programme and he is ready to start his work. My voice is getting little bit quiet for a while till Devendra and Ankita both enjoy this moment of relaxation. The moment of relaxation with full wisdom and ready to put it on the computer he has gathered from all his wisdom. Enjoy this moment for a while. And Devendra you are highly intelligent, very capable, wanting to share all your wisdom and so rather than moving with the jet speed, you are moving with the slow steady quiet peaceful river. Flowing with both the banks, with clear water. Seeing those fish play. Seeing the base of the river with those wide stones and you are computing, composing your session on the computer. With very, very simple language that the students will appreciate highly Devendra. And Devendra is extremely happy on this newly acquired wisdom and experiences this wisdom for a while. Yes, Devendra we are very happy with your performance and all the anxiety and all the stress, all the uneasiness has gone away. Far far away to the horizon with your newly acquired quiet, tranquil self. There is impossibility of any stress, any anger. Yes, with the neck being stretched, you can see the red thread on your right hand. Gradually Devendra, yes with surety, with certainty of his performance he is gradually waking up from this wonderful journey that he experienced. He gathered up everything in his *Agnachakra* or in his forehead. In his prefrontal cortex and being so sure and being so sure of himself as I count from 10 to 1. Devendra you are very sure of yourself. You will practice this 4th state of consciousness which you have experienced today. You will expand this state of consciousness which will help you be more creative. Your creativity will expand. In 10 and 9... 9 and 8... and gradually Devendra is returning to his desk and computer keys. With full assurance of being steady in his self, with clear... yes... gradually you are waking up and 8 and 7... 6 and 5... Devendra your eyes are becoming lighter and lighter and you are opening your eyes and being sure of yourself. Awake from anxiety and stress and anger. Flowing like a smooth flow of a river and 6 and 5 and 4... Yes Devendra, with gradual return to your desk and 3 and 2 and 1. With Ankita on the left side and your pet on the right side and with the open eyes you are visualizing your 3rd eye and with the closed eyes also your 3rd eye helps to understand to function and you are so clever, so intelligent, so creative that now with the count of 1 you are fully awake, aware and take a minute... You can stretch both your arms. You can move from side to side, both your arms, and you are fully awake.

Wonderful Devendra and Ankita. We are very proud of you and you can have a sip of water and after a while you are fully awake with the specs on. It so happens that your throat, your mouth, your tongue becomes a little dry. With this sip of water you will feel very comfortable, quiet within and wake up completely. Thank you very much Devendra and Ankita for taking both of us on this journey of yours. Thank you.

And if you have any questions, please ask.

Session 3

Take out your specs and put them by the side. As Devendra has taken out the specs, he will shed all the anger as easily as he has taken out the specs. Very nice, you have already closed your eyes.

Devendra has already closed his eyes and as he feels his eyes close, and now he tries to open them and there is a familiar feeling already descending on his eyelids. On his eyelids there is a familiar feeling that his eyelids are getting heavier and heavier and still heavier. The light in the room that Devendra and Ankita are sitting is wavering between brighter and still brighter and immediately goes down and that way the relaxation... Dev let your whole body relax. Dev let your whole body relax so much so that even your hair on the head, even the hair that were standing up have settled down. Feel a feeling of settling down all over your body. All over your body and Dev is feeling so nice, so calm. Yes, it is alright to move a little here or there where there is comfort. That tingling has also gone away. Devendra has known this and he has done it a few times before. So easy for him to shut of all the noises, all the sound except my voice and Devendra is now tuning, has already tuned, Devendra is tuning to listen to my voice and as well as his own heart's sounds. His own heart sounds, how nice, how rhythmical, perfectly in a gentle poise. Devendra, this is your gift that nature has given you a heart and that heart has constantly produced this sound that now sounds like a sweet music. Listen to the sweet music of your heart. And be prepared to have a further delightful surprise, Rajni and Bhaskar Vyas, we are privileged to be your friends and so today I have a wonderful choice being offered; be prepared to have the choicest of all choices, the sweets and the food you like the most and that aroma, aroma of the sweet perfume of the choicest food being cooked in your own kitchen. Take a deep, deep breath. Take a deep, deep breath and Dev, deeper still and when you feel the fine fragrance of your choicest food, show me the sacred thread that you have tied on your right hand. Yes. Yes. And that sweet smell has permeated each and every cell of your body. Dev, how nice, how comfortable, how much calm, cool, composed you are. Stay in this calm, cool, composed state when Rajni and I want you to take for a further delightful treat.

Yes, move your head the way you make it more comfortable. Deeper and deeper breath still and be prepared to have further delight and in a wonderful company with Ankita and Devendra have mounted, seated comfortably in the car and Devendra is starting the car engine with his right hand. Yes that sound is not noticed because engine is totally silent but Devendra has started driving the car and he would like to go to a very pleasant even more serene, more silent, perfect solitude of a garden and look, there is a garden. Yes, Devendra, right before your closed eyes, you are parking. You have parked your car perfectly alright. When you park your car to adjust your head, whatever way you like now because you have loosened the seatbelt and you are stepping into a wonderful garden. The garden that you have chosen as a perfectly peaceful, quiet, sweet, serene solitude. Sweet, serene, solitude of a garden and the sun would have risen by now in the east but the sun is a big ball of fire and this fire, this energy is available to Dev as tied by a sacred, sacred thread on his right wrist but that big ball of energy that Dev has tied on his right wrist is only visible to Dev. Yes. See that big ball of energy that you have controlled and relax. Relax. Relax. Relax even more, a further deep, deep breath. When Devendra may like even to further roll down in the chair, he may do so. Roll down in the chair so that your head is comfortable and the sun is hidden behind the clouds in the East but as Devendra relaxes and slides down and if you like you may even lie down. Devendra is so much more comfortable now. Devendra is so much more comfortable now that he has allowed himself the most poignantly poised comfortable position to enjoy the delightful delight of this garden. There is wonderful garden full of flowers that Devendra is seeing as violet. Devendra is seeing violet flowers side by side with some flowers with indigo, blue and violet, indigo and blue flowers are finely, finely like a decorated flower vase or a bouquet are also having some green, green, green leaves. See the green leaves decorating the violet, indigo and blue flowers. What a wonderful delight. What a wonderful garden this is that there are yellow flowers, surrounded by orange flowers as well and the orange flowers are side by side with red flowers also. The red flowers that would be the colour had there not been clouds, the sun also would have been shining so bright now. This spectrum of flowers is side by side. Devendra is so lucky to see a grasp vine and as Devendra is looking at the grapevine, he is now seeing, Devendra is now seeing a fully blown rainbow. What a wonderful delight is this that this rainbow is covering almost the entire panorama of the sky. Wonderful colours of rainbow and the grapevine that Dev is now holding. Dev has started climbing on the grapevine and Dev is taking one step that is 24th July 2022. And as Dev takes further up steps one by one by one, Dev is going up on the grapevine of time so that the year 2023 is yet to come but Dev has yet taken one step backwards to go to 2021 and everything, every occasion, every negative feeling, every kind of monetary loss, every kind of estranged relationships, they come in quick succession; all one at a time. 2021, 2020, 2019, 2018, 2017, 2016, 2015, how quick, how intelligent, how brilliant is Dev to be covering so many events all at once and he wants to proceed further and further up on the rainbow with the help of the grapevine. The grapevine that is time is now showing 2015, 2014, 2013, 2012, 2011, when Dev was getting angry. Of course he was getting angry at that time as well. And so 2012, 2011, 2010 and take a deep, deep breath. You are now high on the rainbow and all the leaves on the grapevine, all the leaves on the grapevine that have shrivelled up, dried, withered away, they are plucked off by Devendra and thrown away onto the Earth from the rainbow. And they are engulfed and burnt out. Devendra is seeing the burning fire, fire that is burning as a quick sudden blaze out of shrivelled and dried leaves of negative feelings. That's such a wonderful work. But Devendra, you have covered something like fourteen years in fourteen minutes and that is really wonderful work. Would you like to go all the way? All the way that once upon a time you were a little baby of about 2 years. If you like to go all the way to your infantile age show me, show me the band. (ID Response - Yes) Okay. Thank you. And I along with Rajni, I am entirely dedicated to Devendra who has now so much work to do. He has taken over the responsibility of Ankita and additionally Ankita has a job and Ankita has a responsibility to maintain the house and there are 2 cats and a dog and 2 infants that are little lovely daughters. So proud of you. Rajni and Bhaskar are so very proud of you that you are wanting to work hard and work hard so as to cover a further period of some 15 or 18 years. We go back to the grapevine. Dev is climbing the grapevine of time backwards and mounting on a rainbow and from 2010 a further step, a further step that will amount to a giant leap... that will amount to a giant leap backwards on the grapevine of time so that in this giant leap, Dev has plucked over several further dried, shrivelled up, useless, colourless, almost so brown as to be turning nearly black, that kind of dried, useless leaves. Dev, throw them down... throw them down.. Again, put them into the blazing fire that is there and as the leaves are dropping further down, the fire is burning bright. See the bright burning fire where you have extinguished and destroyed all those dried and shrivelled negative feelings for more than a decade and now if Devendra is wanting to work even more... Devendra this is so wonderful and this is so much of hard work, it can be tiresome also. So, if you like, tell me whether you are willing to do some more work, show me your right wrist. (ID response - Yes) Okay, I am happy that Devendra wants to go all the way... all the way to the age when he was two years old. Let us pause. Let us rest a while and let us take a deep... deep... deep breath so that with one more giant leap onto this grapevine of time, backwards. The grapevine is taking Devendra further on to the rainbow. Brilliant colours, violet, indigo, blue, extending orange, yellow extending even to bright red and then merging even to white. The rainbow is very much there... very much there all the time but sometimes when it turns white, you don't see it. And there Devendra is seeing a little child, a toddler of Devendra, a toddler that Dev is. Two years... About two years of age... Innocent. A little boy, a toddler walking on both the knees and both the elbows. The toddler is roaming all over the mother earth. Innocent and totally forgetful that whatever leaves he had thrown there into the fire have burnt themselves out. Devendra, my little child. The innocent toddler child of two years. Stay in your pristine innocent poise and stay in this innocent state totally forgetful of all that deserved to be burnt away and have already evaporated into a thin air and now it is my duty along with Dr. Rajni to give you some sweet dreams. We have plucked out several, several dried, shrivelled out leaves of the grapevine. But now we have deserved ourselves to pluck and taste... to pluck and to taste the real sweet grapes that the grapevine of time has. You are seeing how many good, well ripe, seedless grapes. The big grapes that are totally seedless and we see and pluck every grape that this grapevine has borne on itself right from the age that Dev was a toddler till the today. Yes Dev don't be in a hurry. Take your time to sit and taste every delightful grape that the grapevine of time from toddler age 2 Dev is now going to age 3... age 4... he sees himself in a nursery school and age 7 where he is now in a primary school. The primary school that has such a large playground and on the playground there are swings and Dev is enjoying swinging on the swing. How nice... How nice. Be comfortable Dev... you are on a swing and you are certainly not going to fall. You are certainly not going to fall and as the playground and the swings in the playground swing forward and backward, the grapevine takes you forward... the grapevine of the time takes you forward to age 8... 9... 10... 11... 12... and how brilliantly you have performed in your studies. You have enjoyed playing in the school ground and a further leap will take Dev forward... forward... 13... 14... 15... 16... 2016 and everything good and everything nice so that one further leap from 2016, a few years forward gets Devendra married to Ankita. Devendra has such a wonderful, joyful, delightful and pleasant company of a lifetime companion that Ankita is and Ankita's parents... Ankita's father is so affectionate, caring, loving and what a family... what a delightful family this is. Dev it is your 100% well earned and your deserved...

well deserved choice to be happy now. Stay in this happy state... all the dried and shrivelled and withered away leaves on the grapevine have disappeared. Even their smell is gone and even the ash has flown away. So stay in this well deserved state of happiness and enjoy being further progressive... progress in a professional way so that you can support your extended family of 2 cats, and dog and Ankita and yourself. Listen to Dr. Rajni Vyas, she also wants to share your happiness and pleasure and wants your speedy progress. Devendra you have worked so hard that for a while you enjoy this peaceful, quiet, tranquil state for couple of minutes. You had a wonderful journey and take it easy. Stay quiet, calm, comfortable in the position that you are. You enjoy this different type of sleep and rest very, very comfortably. Yes. Your eyes are still heavy so let them rest and enjoy this comfort. Keep lying for a while and you can relax and go to sleep for a while.

Unexplained Reproductive Failure

The following are a set of introductory sessions:

1.

When the investigations are done, and they are all normal, but pregnancy is not occurring so we turn to mind-body connection. There is a close relationship between the mind and the physical body.

When we decide to go ahead with discussion about mind-body connection let us make it sure from both the partners that none of them have any reservations. If they have, let us reveal them without any hesitation. Maybe you would like to think for couple of days that you are sure that you want to reveal your unconscious and sort it out or you need the help of therapist.

Really speaking, in the brain, mind has no position. On the other hand, it is so very interesting that each and every cell has a mind. It sounds so paradoxical to our own mind but studying after 40 long years, we could find out this connection that we divided into three groups. One was a conflict situation which all of us have in small amount or large amount. Conflict always is there. Most of the time we are able to resolve and move forward. We see in little detail about the understanding of conflict. The second group is fear. Everybody has, again, this psychological profile and it is said that there is a chicken in the heart. And third group is intense desire to have a child and results in hyper-anxiety and there is the disturbance in the parameters of hormones, biochemistry, even we have seen the sperms which have been ejected in the vagina in posterior fornix and the mouth of the womb that is cervix. Either they are as if not there because they have been liquefied by the normal content of vagina or they are lying dead or they are various types of movements of the sperms in the pool that we will examine from the vaginal discharge that we will see later.

Now, we see the first group and I would request you in whichever you yourself feel that there is profile, you might just pick it out and then we will have a solution. Starting from the conflict. Now a days there is equal sharing of education, job profile, and all the jobs that a man can do, a lady can do it. There is only one thing that man cannot be the mother. It's only the privilege of a lady to get pregnant and carry the child for 9 months and deliver at the end of 9 months, +/- 10 days. So in conflict, first we will see is the educational disparity. There is a major role that lady has to fulfil of running the house, managing the family and in addition being educated is doing a job. When this additional job work comes up, it is drain on her time and she has to manage not only the time schedule but so many other cultural situations have to be managed by a lady and we found it to be a point of stress. Second thing is the economical disparity. One of the partners is economically better off and it comes in the interpersonal relationship of the couple. Either from the family one is higher up or a lady is earning better than the husband because culturally it is acceptable that man is the bread earner and the lady is running the house looking after the family and children. This additional job brings about quite an adjustment, understanding between the couple as well as the family. Family's expectations are very high from a daughter in law and have to accept that she is educated and doing a job as well.

The third is the cultural disparity. Till few decades back, it was intercaste marriage which was to be adjusted for but now it is not only intercaste but even international. And so there is so much of cultural difference than that in love marriages as it is said, 'marry in hurry, and repent at leisure'. In between this hurry and repent, so many levels occur. And in planning the child this comes as a big controversy. The fourth is professional disparity or discord. Maybe one of the partners is higher up in earning or in position and the other partner has all the time issue in the mind. When we are talking such conflicting situation, in the beginning of our journey, it was very difficult to understand; after couple of interviews, gradually these situations was a big issue and when resolved we got the good result. Taking this forward, there is a career expectation also. Joining in a lower grade, waiting for promotion, maybe one may not come up as per expectation, and then the frustration starts as to when I will become a boss or when I will earn still better. And so many times we found that there was a postponement of planning a child. It so happened that in the beginning the lady might or both the partners might feel that it is too early to plan a child. Now a days late marriages and expectation of the career, we observed that 30 is the right age, maybe plus minus two or three years. So that, by the time the child is 20, the parents are around 50. Couples have come and asked us what is the right age to plan the child and this has been our standard advice of 30 plus or minus 2. Though, now we have observed that fertility is quite efficient till the age of 45-47 but then the child is too young when the parents are nearing retiring age. If it is by age of 30, the child grows up and is about to be finishing the education and settling for a job. There are so many plus and minus advantage and disadvantages but of long experience we have seen that this is the right age. Postponing of the pregnancy results in so many situations and conflicts in the mind of a couple. Now, the joint family is getting less and less, but still in joint family, the lady is at a disadvantage and there is quite some discord and dominance of the seniors and has to comply and adjust which is a cause of conflict. She feels that at the moment when she is not able to adjust. Once there is a child it would be still more difficult. Even if it's not a joint family, mother in law is quite an issue in the relationship of a couple. Once sorted out, it moves quite smooth. The extreme example which I took time to understand, I would like to narrate.

Usually, in the past, mother in law and daughter in law used to come and then after 3 or 4 interviews I said, 'Now, I will need husband to come.' The mother in law blurted out that, 'I am coming, why do you need him?' I said, 'I have to understand.' And then she was in rage. And next time I told I want a semen examination and a semen sample, is it possible that if he does not come, it is a test that I can do?' She understood the need of the couple. The daughter in law has said previously that she is a bird in a golden cage and I was surprised to listen to the detail and such situations may not be very common but it is possible. So many times we have asked the couple, who wants the child? The lady, the husband or the family?' and we have got various answers which were tackled and here also a couple approached us for infertility and the husband sits and before I could even start my interview, he says, 'I have been telling my wife, lets adopt. Why have the botheration of undergoing all this? If we go to buy a shirt, we shop around 3 or 4 shops and buy a shirt. So we can go in the orphanage, maybe 2 or 3 and just have a child.' Such shocks we used to get in the interview and couples went on moving from pillar to post that they are infertile.

The next was second marriage. Maybe the first marriage has a child or has a bad experience and so many such causes and they were wondering and postponing to have a child and hostility either to the partner or to their families. So such 10 causes we found in the causation of conflict.

So I would request whether you have any of such conflicting situations, maybe you can sort it out between two of you or take our help to sort out. It's not very difficult. The fact that you have agreed to be the partners in life and now wanting to have a child, these conflicting situations can be just sorted out either by talking it out or deleting it in hypnosis.

The second group is of fear. Fear of what?

It's very interesting. A lady is afraid to lose her charm, to lose her figure, to lose her personality or to carry a pregnancy for 9 months and when it was explained that every moment in the world, one child is born. It is the way of nature that the world goes on, on the birth whether they are human beings or animals or going up to all kinds of live beings including insects. Certain things when told come as knowledge with surprise that we have not looked around at all. Sometimes earlier abortions or abortion is a fear. We have treated a lady with 10 abortions having a full time child as the 11th pregnancy. Maybe there is a cause for abortion and then it's treated or just taking her forward assuring her all the time, investigating that the child that she is carrying is absolutely normal and has gone to term. Two or three abortions have been common in our observation. Fear of child bearing, carrying and rearing, all this is a phenomenon which is really a natural phenomenon but assurance is required at any stage and after the birth of the child, carrying her for all 9 months with frequent visits, assurances and hypnosis ultimately she completely broke down and lost a child on 15th day because she was afraid to lose the job. Second time when she became pregnant, we took the assurance from the people with whom she was working that she would be given three months holidays. Now this situation is getting less because companies have agreed to give six months to one year of holiday and even paternal leave. So many times, the mother has brought the daughter, or the mother in law has brought the daughter in law saying that there is a family history of sterility so please treat her within six months of marriage and see that she becomes pregnant and doesn't get aborted and so on and so forth. It is not transmitted from generation to generation and assurances have been quite sufficient. Going on the Google and reading the physiology and understanding from the Google who usually says on both the sides, there is fear of pain, abortion, deformed child, etc. When the physiology is read, and the abdomen becomes big and the uterus stretches and then the foetus grows and so on and so and the there will be pain of the delivery and the description, usually they are afraid and the answer is same. They are natural phenomena and if need be elective caesarean section is available. As we discussed before, 30 years is the right age for having a child. There has been a late age of marriage also. When there is a late age of marriage, people have many fears of congenital malformation, of them being old and having complications of age related diseases like diabetes or blood pressure and so many other fears of rearing the child. Usually, the assurance worked out and we have quite a few elderly ladies who had normal pregnancy and a normal child. Previous caesarean section or ectopic pregnancy also is the fear complex. Now a days early diagnosis of ectopic pregnancy and saving the tube without removing the tube. Minimum three sections are possible though we have observed five caesarean sections though we had to be extremely careful in the antenatal and intranatal period. Illness of one of the partners of any kind, we have to assure for having a normal child. Previous congenitally deformed child is also a cause of fear and during this pregnancy, modern investigations like sonography and amniotic fluid study can rule out this congenital deformity. This way the fear has to be found out and then fear that we have diagnosed has to be tackled accordingly. So if you have any of such reservations, please identify and sort it out with your obstetrician.

The third group has been the intense desire. Listening to the history and stories of friends and family and relations, there is intense desire. A lady can become pregnant once a month because she ovulates once a month. Out of 12 months, maybe 1 month she may not ovulate, so maybe it is 11 months. The man has sperms less or more all round the year. That also can fluctuate from 0 to any number. One of the stock market broker said that my sperm count fluctuates with the NSE, BSE index. So I need not emphasize that mind and body are one and they influence each other. Way back Sushrut said, 'Pragnyaaparadha Jayate Sarva Rogaan'. In short saying that when your intellect is affected, it is at that time that mind-body connection gets affected in so many ways. So this intense desire of hyper anxiety and agitation has so many repercussions on hormones, biochemistry, molecular biology, sperms, ovum, ovulation and so on. Traditionally and all over the world we have seen that there is very few percentage who wants a child while most of the time male child is preferred. There are various reasons and various explanations that are given and I am sure that you know that sex determination came in a big way in the 90s when so many abortions occurred and it was female foeticide and the government had to stop the sex determination and now it is not allowed. And very important and when we realized this cause, we were at a loss. And that was a high ideal for a child to be born; has to be intelligent like Einstein, has to be handsome like Amitabh Bachchan, has to be absolutely a handsome little one. They have forgotten the genetics. It is not only the genes but so many other factors which affect the child. Maybe you might have some other doubts; which I would request, that please sort it out with your obstetrician and have no doubt to become the parent of a child.

Thank you very much for your patient listening.

Thank you.

2.

This script is for understanding about Mind-Body connection.

It may be that some time in this talk there might be a repetition but this is for emphasizing certain points which is important for understanding Mind-Body connection. Usually, right from the time of our primary school, we have learnt the 1+1 =2 and 2+2 =4. The computer also works on this principle and in the mind now recently it has been established that Mind-Body connection is such because there are so many hormones, so many biochemical substances that are produced in the body. So much interplay between all these substances, hormones and the body fluids. Memory and the result is that in the body 1+1 becomes 2, 4 and you can add and make it plus or it might become minus instead of plus 2, when we add 1+1 it may become -2, -200, -2000. And so, each individual has the same physical body but emotional body, the mind, the brain, is very different and can you believe that this mind in 24 hours, has something like 60,000 thoughts going through this time. Believe me, when I heard for the first time, I wondered how they would have counted, and you all have an answer that it is the computer. When you are listening to me, each and every word that I speak, you listen and analyze and what we call at the back of the mind, you wonder what I am talking is sense or nonsense. This is what each and every human being experiences and it is this experience of the 4th state about which we are going to talk about. We understand that it is neither awake nor dreaming, nor sleep because the mind is not there and so to verbalize this 4th state onwards upto the 7th state is not easily verbalized but this is what we call as experiential. So in many ways it is described that the experience was out of the world, or stayed 0 or meditative state or *Samadhi*. So, I would like to make you understand because mind always wants to understand but mind does not experience unless you keep on practicing. There are various relaxation sessions that you will come across. If you believe in deities you can visualize the deities, if not, because nowadays this is a common parlance that I don't believe in God. Yes, there is something, but not God. Ok. Again the same thing, the individual wants to do something different.

So, in this creative visualization also, we can be on a sea beach and be one with the waves coming in a tide and horizon where sea and sky meets. Or coming from mountains people can be on mountains, Himalayas and valleys or be with the Nature. Maybe a beautiful flower or a singing bird or any of the pleasant memory that you have and you get lost and you wake up and wonder how much the time has passed.

So we are going to talk something about this. In our experience most of the things that happens, happens in this state because mind has conscious, subconscious and unconscious levels. This unconscious usually plays a great part in our day to day working behaviour and belief system.

This belief system is also a wonderful thing. So many times we say that, I believe that it is like this and what you believe, I don't agree and vice versa and so many such beliefs are stored in our unconscious and it makes us function on such beliefs. Like black cat is a bad omen and when it turns out to be good because you did not get that bus ride when it was a bad omen but that bus met with an accident. When one starts thinking in this fashion in this scientific world and computer world that you press a button and you can talk at thousands of miles away. It has a scientific explanation but as a joke, 'Ram and Sita did travel in Pushkar aeroplane from Lanka to Ayodhya.' Oh, they are all stories. They are. But today, we do travel in aeroplane all round the world. So, belief system is also very important in our day to day behaviour. But we have hardly any time to think about this. So please think.

I would like to introduce another parameter, what is called as a personality, or a left brain or a right brain. Or a personality A and B type.

A type is analytical, mathematical, very sure about the results, want to work very fast, don't want to be challenged, all the time wanting to be on the top and many more.

While B type is a Hindu wife of olden times who sits and works at home, very quiet, opines if asked, but understands everything. Not very calculative, not very mathematical but enjoys soft side of life like music, painting, nature and so on. So when we will talk about the therapy, you will find out your own personality, whether it is A or B. For more, always computer and Google is available to you.

To accept this mind-body connection is one of the important requirement in this therapy and if one accepts, believes, imbibes, we have seen the result coming in 2-3 months or in a very short time. People who is a closed system, who is not ready for a change, it takes little longer depending upon their acceptability and not keeping the doors closed of their minds and making the mind a friend and ask to sit by side and not keep on arguing against to get good results.

Taking the challenge that what you are telling, I don't believe may be you may not go further or try and listen the cassettes and people in our experience have changed their approach, their attitude and their itch to know better and in that, might go into the 4th state of consciousness and that is *Turya.*

This short note will make you go further and further in our session one by one. And believe me, in modern scientific computer world; to believe that there is something called 4th state of consciousness, requires open mind and acceptability.

Thank you very much for this patient hearing and now you can go to the introduction of our cassettes and few figures and let me tell you that if you have accepted what Mind-Body connection can do and if destiny is in your favour, you will be rewarded with a valuable, beautiful gift of nature. You are lucky to have such a wonderful gift which is due to you both and best of luck from Drs. Vyas.

Thank you very much for patient hearing

3.

Friends, today we will understand the basic anatomical structure of the genital tract. There is a vagina in which part of the uterus called cervix is projecting and the rest of the uterus is in the lower part of the tummy. Uterus has the upper part called fundus, below are the tubes on either sides. There is body of the uterus. It lowers down into the internal os, that is the beginning of cervix which is 1 inch long is external os which projects into the vagina.

This uterus size is something like the size of a fist which is about 10 cm. But, it grows right up to the diaphragm and when the baby is at the full term, it stretches to accommodate 5-7 pounds of the foetus, about 1 and half litre of water and around 1 and a half pound of placenta. It is that stretchability, then again after delivery from 6 weeks to 3 months, uterus comes back to normal size. As we will talk further and further, you will realize how the nature has made each and every part of the body to the whole nature in such a way that it keeps on working of its own without our knowing at the conscious level. This uterus has outside peritoneum, then there is thick musculature, the inner lining is endometrium. This endometrium grows from 1 mm to 10 mm every month and the menstruation occurs during 28-32 days. Most of the time it is regular and this cycle goes on from the adolescence to menopause. That means it works for about 35 years to 40 years and it can produce each and every year, 1 baby. But we want only one or two at the most so that these two babies, when they grow up as adults, has support of each other and the life goes on. This is so mechanical on one hand and so we let nature work. Not worry about understand or worry about anything. Surrender to nature and it will just happen that you have missed the period and pregnancy test is positive. Endometrium grows from 1 to 2 mm and if pregnancy does not occur, it gets shedded off as menstruation. 3-5 days of moderate amount is the normal outflow from shedding from the body of the uterus and comes out from the internal os to external os to vagina and it is the menstrual cycle. This is important to know that when the menstrual period does not occur, it means, it is called amenorrhea and it is most common in married women to be pregnant with this background.

Next we go to vagina and the external os and internal os. Internal os during menstruation opens up and during delivery the external and internal os completely widely opens, becomes almost one and the baby descends and the delivery occurs from the vagina. It is described as a elephant walking out of a keyhole. When we think of such a natural phenomenon, and every second in the world, the delivery occurs and newborn is born and you wonder how, and since ages the world keeps on reproducing and the cycle goes on. We have no time to even think as to how the nature has been performing years after years.

Now let us know another action of the cervix. When the intercourse occurs through the vagina, there is deposition of semen onto the external os and there is a pull in the upper part of the vagina. This upper part of the vagina allows so many sperms to enter into the cervix and it goes from the external os through the internal os, body of the uterus and so many sperms enter into the uterus through the tube and they go into the tube to meet the ovum which we will see when we talk about ovary and the conception occurs in the tube and gradually it moves in 4 to 5 days into the uterus and settles for 9 months and 10 days, which is a normal time for the baby to be fully grown, completely with a physical body and all the internal controls and this baby grows into the adult that you are.

This is the normal part of the uterus and now we get connected with the endocrinologist part where the follicular stimulating hormone starts secreting on the first day and this follicular stimulating hormone, stimulates the ovary and 4-5 ovum gets stimulated. The ovary contains something like 30,000 ova and so if allowed naturally to grow, there is always ova available for conception. 4-5 ovas which is in size of a µ (Mu), that is thousandth of 1 millimetre grows and it grows to 2 centimetres. Usually, there is what is called as a dominant follicle and usually out of 4 to 5, one becomes dominant follicle and between 12th to 14th day, this two centimetre ovum bursts and the ova comes out. This when it grows to 2 centimetres, it has a lining that secretes what is called as estrogen which goes to endometrium to grow from the baseline to something like 8-10 millimetre size. It is very juicy and it is here that ultimately the conceived ovum settles down and it becomes a baby. So the chances of pregnancy usually in human beings is between 12-14 days and so that is the time that intercourse is must on alternate day. Otherwise during month couple can decide for themselves about intercourse. This ovum lives for about 24 hours. so in a year, usually a woman ovulates only 12 times and may be because of stresses, situations, once in a month ovulation may not occur. As ovulation does not occur, so 10-11 times lady can become pregnant in a year.

While in men, it is different all round the year sperms are there in semen. Sometimes more and sometimes less. As share market broker has described that when SENSEX is high, sperm count is high. When SENSEX falls, the count is low. This conveys its relationship with stress. Sometimes it is more, sometimes it is less depending upon so many factors. But woman can become pregnant in a month once. While man can deposit semen all round the year. So record of 100 children to a man with many wives!!!! During pregnancy there is no ovulation. Ovulation is suppressed.

Coming back to follicle stimulating hormone which has stimulated this ovary and oestrogen which sends the message to say that 2 cm or 2.1 cm and so naturally FSH stops secreting and the next hormone is secreted by pituitary what is called as luteinizing hormone. This hormone is a very sensitive hormone and in medical terms it is called a pulsatile hormone. And this is a very important time for a lady for ovulation who was to become pregnant. Any stress, any situation and this luteinizing hormone goes haywire. We restrict at the moment for the normal cycle and so FSH level goes down and LH level comes up releases and the 2.1 cm ovum burst and ova is liberated. This is picked up by the tube which has prongs which sits on to that ova and takes and brings about into the tube. When so many sperms enter through the os, and meets the ova, only one ova and one sperm makes the baby. Then why we worry when there are less sperms? Only one sperm is required, the rest of them liquefy and make the surrounding more favourable, so that sperm can enter ova-zona pellicuda. This ruptured ova collapses and then starts producing hormone from pituitary called progesterone which makes endometrium more juicy, more lively and it prepares the bed for conceived ova and the conceived ova comes and settles into the uterus. It becomes very receptive and continues which ultimately makes a baby to settle, to be born after 9 months. The ruptured cyst continues to grow and secretes progesterone. The progesterone helps endometrium grow further, more blood supply occurs. It increases in thickness, becomes more velvety and juicy. It prepares itself for nidation of blastocyst which travels from tube and settles in uterus. It stays there for 9 months and 10 days. In the conceived ovum takes over the secretion and the placenta is formed which will nourish the baby for the rest of the time. So this is in short how the conception and the pregnancy occurs remains into the house of uterus.

One of my friends told me a story that a boy whom she had delivered said that today my mother sold off my original house and she was wonderstruck and asked him, he said that my mother's uterus is removed which was my first home. So, this is what the feeling is for the foetus for 9 months and 10 days which is the usual normal count. And this is the normal cycle which is in the form of W. From the pituitary, follicular stimulating hormone, which is FSH comes into the circulation and stimulates the ovary, ovary in turn has an ovum which starts growing and one becomes a dominant follicle and then it secretes estrogens which after 13 days goes and tells that now I am grown up and then this luteinizing hormone is secreted by pituitary, it ruptures and brings out from that grown ovum to be picked up by the fimbiral end of the fallopian tube and the conception occurs. LH is secreted for few days and this ruptured ovum is sealed off and continues to secrete what is called as progesterone which helps ultimately to form the placenta. If pregnancy does not occur as we discussed after 28-32 days depending on the individual, the menstruation occurs and this cycle goes on during child bearing age, about age of 13-45. So, you can imagine how many children you can produce. But, we want 2 children and the interval between the two can be kept as 2 years so that the mother's health is regained completely to bear another child while this child is grown to 2 years and is self-sufficient and she can have a second child. This cycle is a normal cycle in human beings and as you know that even after rape, the conception can occur. So conception is a wonder of the world on one hand and on the other hand you go to see, it keeps on occurring. As I said, every minute a child is born in this world. So you can see that it is very natural, very normal for all the living beings to procreate and the world goes on. In animals, it is different and there is a mating season and when they mate, at that time, the ovulation occurs. So you can have an explanation that most of the time, 12-15 days is the period for conception for a human being but there is always an exception and it can occur at anytime of the month may be imitating an animal. This is the normal human cycle and so we have to allow this rhythm of W as FSH, oestrogen, LH and progesterone to occur because this is one of the most sensitive hormones which are easily affected by stress. Let the river flow, the same way, let the hormones flow and as the hormones flow in its own way, the pregnancy is very, very easy to happen.

The following figure will help you to understand the process of fertilization better:

THE INTRICATE PROCESS OF FERTILIZATION

For fertilization to occur, a single egg and millions of sperm are produced and egg sperm meet in a carefully timed intricate process. In the woman, an egg is released (ovulation) once in each cycle at approximately 28 days. In the man, sperm are continuously produced in 90-day cycles. At ejaculation, up to 500 million sperm are released and must swim through the vagina, cervix, and uterus to meet the egg in the fallopian tube within hours of ovulation. The process is so intricate that even the most fertile couple has only a one in four chance of conceiving each month.

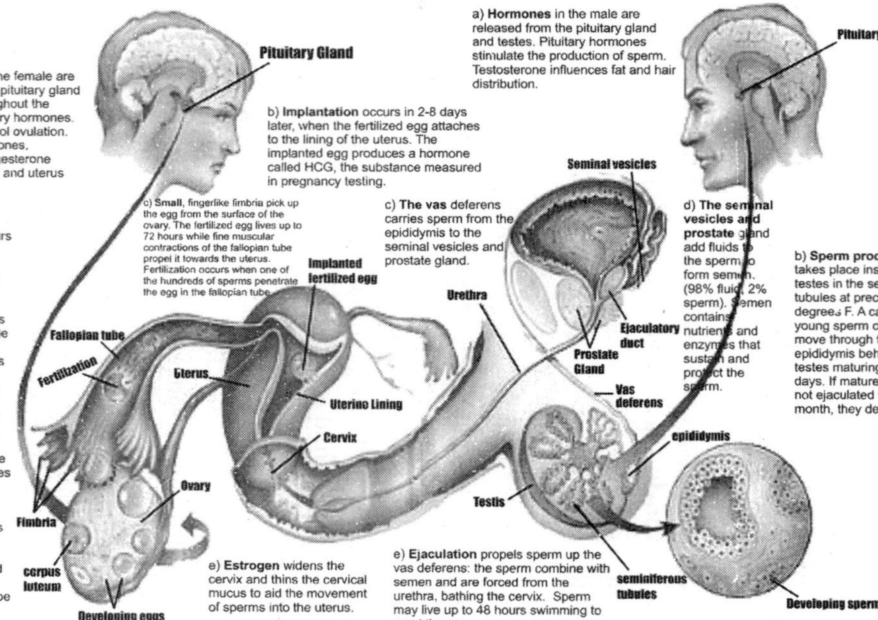

a) **Hormones** in the female are released from the pituitary gland and ovaries throughout the month. The pituitary hormones. FSH and LH control ovulation. The ovarian hormones, estrogen and progesterone prepare the cervix and uterus for conception.

b) **Ovulation** occurs once a month at mid-cycle. Eggs begin to mature in either ovary in response to FSH. Each egg develops a bubble-like follicle which produces increased amounts of estrogen. The estrogen prepares the cervix and cervical mucus for the passage of sperm. It also triggers the release of LH, which causes the mature egg to be released from the ovary. After ovulation, a corpus luteum is formed. Progesterone is then produced and an elevated temperature may be recorded.

c) **Small**, fingerlike fimbria pick up the egg from the surface of the ovary. The fertilized egg lives up to 72 hours while fine muscular contractions of the fallopian tube propel it towards the uterus. Fertilization occurs when one of the hundreds of sperms penetrate the egg in the fallopian tube.

b) **Implantation** occurs in 2-8 days later, when the fertilized egg attaches to the lining of the uterus. The implanted egg produces a hormone called HCG, the substance measured in pregnancy testing.

e) **Estrogen** widens the cervix and thins the cervical mucus to aid the movement of sperms into the uterus.

a) **Hormones** in the male are released from the pituitary gland and testes. Pituitary hormones stimulate the production of sperm. Testosterone influences fat and hair distribution.

c) **The vas** deferens carries sperm from the epididymis to the seminal vesicles and prostate gland.

d) **The seminal vesicles and prostate** gland add fluids to the sperm to form semen. (98% fluid, 2% sperm). Semen contains nutrients and enzymes that sustain and protect the sperm.

b) **Sperm production** takes place inside the testes in the seminiferous tubules at precisely 94 degrees F. A cascade of young sperm continually move through the coiled epididymis behind each testes maturing for 12 days. If mature sperm are not ejaculated within a month, they deteriorate.

e) **Ejaculation** propels sperm up the vas deferens: the sperm combine with semen and are forced from the urethra, bathing the cervix. Sperm may live up to 48 hours swimming to meet the egg.

4. Ovulation

We have discussed the process of ovulation when we discussed physiology. We will repeat in context of sonography as well as Hypnotherapy.

On the 4th day of menstrual cycle for base line Sonography will be done. This time will see 3 to 5 follicles of size 3 to 4 mm. The follow up will be on 8th or 9th day. Preferably the lady will not see the report. She will be asked by sonographer to come on alternate day or daily depending on growth of follicle. Usually it ruptures between 13th to 15th day. It varies with individual.

The session that is given now is rupture of follicle and conception.

DP and DV, two days ago we have done the relaxation exercise and you have also tried to this relaxation at home. We have tried a different route as well. Taking in a deep breath and exhaling, relax your body. Relax. Take a deep breath. Deep breath. In and out. Wonderful!

Take a deep breath, in and out and as you take that deep breath in, to take that oxygenated energized, universally around you which exists, which at the time of birth till today you have been breathing and that is an important... very, very important life source. This has been happening without your knowledge, with your knowledge and you have done it so many times. To count will require the help of a computer. You breathe in and out every minute 14 to 18 times in one minute. That is multiplied by 60 times then by 24 times then by 365 then by your age. So, you are so much... so much accustomed... It's a habit and it just happens automatically. The same way your heart and the same way you are taking food. So these are all natural processes. It's a birthright. You've done it and you can do it. The same way you have grown up. You are married. It's your birthright to have a child. It has to happen as you relax, start relaxation from the sole of your feet. Yes DP... Yes... both of you are wonderful creations of God. We want to create one such wonderful creation, taking shape from both of you. As you relax. As you open up all your doors, this relaxation wave from ankles goes to both your legs, back and front. Then to your knees and to the bulky muscles of your thighs. They pass the weight of the upper body to the knees and to the ground and makes you active and moving always forward. Let them relax and let the fresh, energized, oxygenated blood into your legs, knees, thighs and take away all that used carbon dioxide and all that toxic material through the blood and it goes out from your system as you breathe out. Wonderful. Very nice. Let that... that wave of relaxation move up in your tummy.

That wonderful Pandora box contains so many things, so many organs which function as normally as your breathing. As your heart works regularly, rhythmically, constantly, not for a second does it stop, the same way all the organs in your abdomen also work the same way. It is described as a biological clock. That biological clock knows what it has to do. It functions normally, rhythmically as the sun rises in the East at certain time. As it sets at a certain time, it has a regular cycle. The same way the moon, being a reflected glory of the sun goes full moon and finishes its cycle. These are all biological... all natural laws... that Almighty which is present every moment, every second, every minute. His presence, you can experience, you can feel, you can see with the mental eyes in your brain. He regulates wonderfully this cycle. This biological clock... let it function normally, regularly... DV and DP have given over the charge to regulate, to work according to the laws of nature that Almighty knows and have completely surrendered to that unseen. The ordinary eyes can be seen, mental eyes can be felt, can be heard by that 'Anahad naad' can be smelled with a fine fragrance of your choice around you. Just feel His presence and observe Him working and if you can feel His presence or you can see with your mental eyes, please let me know. Coming very, very gently, very affectionately, very lovingly and is pouring all the blessings. Agreeing to do all that is necessary. You have made a space in your heart and in your brain. You have done what is described in our scriptures as 'Praan Pratishtha'. In your heart and in your brain you are feeling His presence all over your body. Each and every cell is singing, is dancing and making DP and DV joyful in fantasy.

Please enjoy these moments and fill it up in each and every nook and corner, each and every cell of your body. Kabir says, 'Kan Kan mein hi panchi bolta'. Each and every cell of your body has a mind and is functionung in rhythmic fashion. Let every moment enjoy His presence, His singing, His blessings, His caring, His love, and His affection within yourself and in company of each other. DP and DV, please feel and enjoy His presence for few minutes. If you have felt all that please move your respective finger. If you feel the presence of that Almighty which is singing, which is dancing, who is all the time present in each and every cell of your body, please indicate his presence... Yes. Wonderful! Excellent! Yes DP. Please let me know his presence within you if you feel Him singing. If you are visualizing... DP, please let me know. Also let me know whether you would like to move forward. Okay... very good, very nice... And as you are visualizing, hearing, smelling, feeling His presence. This is an experience... it is beyond words. The experience that you experience in a moment takes ages to toil to express it. Sri Aurobindo felt this experience, this feeling, this moment of His presence in this very compound where you are there. He felt it, he carried it forward for 45 long years. He was always with him... that Almighty was always within him and he guided him throughout his life. We ask His blessings, His presence at any time, at every time at every moment to guide us, to help us, to run that biological clock that He has fit in us. He always shows the right way. After surrendering Him we can be quiet, peaceful, tranquil, happy, joyful like a child in the mother's lap. It is a wonderful experience... Keep on experiencing this moment without any worries, any tensions, any stress. It is His responsibility to carry on the work our whole existence. All our activities, all these are His responsibilities. Please, for a while feel His presence.

Yes, DP, DV, you have felt His presence, you have heard your own heartbeats. You have heard His divine music you've enjoyed His presence. And once experienced, once surrendered, it is His responsibility to put us on the right path, function in the right, accurate, proper way. He has chalked out our whole programme.

This relaxation goes up into the brain. Into the mind. Whole of the face. He regularizes all the hormones that has to work according to the biological clock. As you are hearing your heartbeats, quietly breathing in... taking all that universal energy, that oxygen, the fresh air, the fragrant air within you. The same way all these hormones also will work as required, as wanted at the time that they are wanted... He is giving full assurance of His full cooperation... all the help... all the help to make it function normally. Hence, Arjun in *Geeta* stays in the 'Rath' where Shri Krishna takes him. The same way DP and DV has handed over the reins to that Almighty who is sitting in their heart and in their brain. How wonderful to feel that peace, that peace, that tranquillity, like a child in the mother's womb. And the same way DP and DV are going to make that soul comfortable in the womb of DP. Visualize His presence DP in your womb as a new creation by DV and DP. Jointly doing a new creation with the help of *Saarthi*, who is guiding the way. If both of you are convinced and only if you are convinced about our victory in the venture that we have taken forwards, sure and if only sure, please indicate to me with your finger DP... .Very nice. Wonderful. Yes DP, if you have handed over the reins to that Almighty, and if you are sure, convinced fully, please indicate me with your finger. Very nice. Wonderful.

He is accepted to take this rein in his hand, it's moving with full responsibility, in full earnestness... full agreement and enjoy his presence for few minutes on this festival of joy, peace, quietness within.

Both of you are fully convinced about our moving forward, just relaxing. Where somebody is driving us in the right path, in the right direction to achieve the right goal. You are fully convinced and feeling all this experience in your heart and in your brain. You wake up fully alert. Assured. Ready to be guided, to be working according to that biological clock to achieve the goal. Wonderful. Any of your endeavours, He will always be present... . Always success is within you... Yes, success is 100% there. Please keep all your drawers, all your windows, all your surroundings open to this vital presence of

Almighty and wake up when you are fully convinced about what I have described to you. What you have visualized, what you have heard, what you have smelled, all his presence which is circulating all over yourself. Yes, DP. Only and only when you are convinced, then you move your finger accordingly. DP, have a full assurance of His presence which you have already felt... where you have already done that 'Praan Prathishtha' in your heart, in your brain. You open your mental eyes, your mental ears, and listen to that 'Anahat Naad' and after that full conviction, when I count from 5 to 1, you wake up.

5.

Friends, today we are going to understand one test which increases the pregnancy rate when this test comes positive. This is known as the post-Coital test and the way it is done is that within half an hour after coitus, you go to the gynaecologist. The gynaecologist aspirates something from external ors and pool of the semen in vagina and sends it to the pathologist. This consumes so much of time that chances of it coming false negative is so high that we could not establish what we wanted to see. So, we have modified this test and this is called as Vyas' modification of post-coital test. Here what we do is that we call the couple to the consulting room and by masturbation, the semen is collected in the bottle and it is brought to the consulting room where the gynaecologist fills up in the AI syringe and with the AI cannula puts this semen in the vagina on external ors and the other part drops into posterior fornix. The lady is asked to lie down for half an hour and then the gynaecologist takes 3 slides. One from the semen that is collected in the bottle, 2nd from the external ors, and the opening of the ors and 3rd from the posterior vaginal pool and sees under the microscope. This was our very interesting observation that the couple howsoever illiterate could see it under the microscope and we had to explain what we have seen. Now positive post-coital test is the sperms that they see in the sample from the bottle, the sperms are running away from the site and this live demonstration thrills the patients. Now, the positive test is that from the ors and the posterior vaginal wall, the sperms are moving with the same speed and so it is easily able to go through external ors, internal ors, to the uterine canal and in the opening of the fallopian tube enters the fallopian tube and the chances of conception is quite high but we saw various results.

What were they?

What we saw was a negative post-coital test and believe me that we were surprised that whether we did put the semen on the cervix and posterior vaginal wall? Because there were no sperms and this indicates that there was a liquification of the semen by the vaginal discharge and after our interpretation and discussion; this is a negative post-coital test where there is so much of resentment and rejection by the partner and there is high incidence of immunity and IgA, IgM and IgG were responsible for this and our fellow colleague has measured this and this is autoimmune.

The second observation was a little less resentment but not very sure and there was a immune reaction where we saw the sperms lying like a dead soldier.

The third was they were very sluggishly moving forward or backwards and this is the interpretation as the doubt in the mind of a lady or even in the man.

The fourth interpretation was they were moving round and round and believe me, when we asked the husband of a lady who was very assertive and aggressive, he said, "Don't you see that I am moving all the time around my wife? But she is what you have seen her." And taking this case further, she decided to give up and she adopted a child of 5 years. She was a high official in the bank. Rose up quite a bit in the position in the bank and came back after 7 years of her adoption and I was surprised. I asked her, "Why have you come?"

She says, "Look at my adopted child. She is 12 years and she is ready to sue me because she says that I am very strict with her and I have threatened her to put back in the orphanage, and because I have adopted legally, she says that she is going to sue me unless I write all my property to her." What a vagary of fate and future. But the interesting thing that I want to draw your attention is that both husband and wife have to be convinced to have a child, will be able to take all the responsibilities with the family, with the help of whatever is needed and plan the child. As we observed and we have analyzed the post-coital test in our paper and we were very happy to correct in such a big number that the patient with negative PC test started coming in 3-4 months to tell us that we have resorted our differences by themselves and see whether the post-coital test is positive. With so many such different experiences, we feel that this test has a high value in the treatment of infertility. You can request the gynaecologist that they might do this test as we have recommended and the result can be seen by yourself and there is a self cure by understanding this phenomena.

So, this is an autoimmune response that is responsible at the level of the vagina but it could also have an effect in the endometrial canal, in the mucosa of tube, and one has to really gather up and understanding between both the partners that they are sure to have a child and success guaranteed.

As we have seen there is this autoimmune reaction, there is a same way hormone imbalance. Particularly when the hormone assessment is done, the LH, being a pulsatile hormone is also affected by psyche and the same way as we have discussed, the man under stress can show from azoospermia to 70-90 milllion of cells on the second test. So, it is very interesting that psychological preparation has to be there and for both the partner, they have to decide that yes, we want to have a nice, beautiful child of our own who would carry on our heritage and then the road is very clear for them.

So, this shows about the post-coital test and its interpretation. The same way about FSH, oestrogen, LH and progestron, the figure of 'W' that we have discussed and another is autonomic nervous system which has to make the parasympathetic system to relax and help the conception to occur after the ovulation and the conception. So, these three factors that we have discussed are very important for normally anatomical and physiological status of both the husband and wife but not conceiving. So, the stress that is there, which we have discussed in various ways should be considered and it has to happen, and it will happen. You have passed such high degree and are working in high position like IT companies or in a bank or anywhere where you are highly intelligent couple but let me tell you that these are 'A' type of personality. 'A' type of personality wants to perform, is calculative, is mathematical, is analytical and wants to have always win and so if you convert this to 'B' type of personality, where there is love, affection, caring, having ideas about painting, music, just be with nature, not calculative, a 'B' type of personality and be a whole brain that is right and left which is necessary to live happily, working happily and you have won the game of happy living. Always in '*Anandmayakosh*'. This is something about post-coital test that we have understood the normal physiology. As you know that after the war, with high incidence of rape occurring, the girl, the woman becomes pregnant and so to become pregnant is a normal, natural phenomenon; as we eat, as we drink and as we live our lives and so go within yourself and ask what is the reservation and success is in front of you.

All the Best for the conception. Thank you very much for patient listening and best of luck.

6.

Friends we studied about the PC test, its interpretation and help in increasing the possibility of conception. Now I will want to add something more about artificial insemination. We process the semen and remove all that is causing this immunological situation and we prepare a semen sample which can be put directly into the uterus. So, we have jumped the cervical mucus which could be the obstacle and the sperms might be dying and this is the scientific explanation. Sometimes we succeed, but quite a few times, it is not only the cervical mucous, it is the genital tract and the body and the lady is still not prepared to be the mother. So, the sperms die and conception does not occur and artificial insemination fails. This is a situation. The same thing is about the IVF.

In IVF, we aspirate the ova and try to put ova and sperms together and see that the conception occurs. After a while, it has reached the stage of blastocyst, 3 or 4 conceived ova are put into the uterus. Even then the incidence of success is 10-15%. Why? It could be an immunological factor where we spoke about IgA, IgM, IgG, etc. which might be the cause in endometrium, in the tube and ultimately it is in the mind because after sorting out the factors that we have already discussed, naturally, it has been observed that woman becomes pregnant without the help of IVF. Why? We have to accept that science is advancing very very fast but all the same, life and death is in the hand of Almighty. Secondly, with psychosomatic medicine having a place, the mind is analyzed extensively by psychologists, philosophers and hypnotherapy. So, when the mind is healthy, mind is without any prejudices, any of the situations which mind has not accepted, whatsoever may be tried, and it fails. So we are discussing all these factors and take into consideration the mind having a great say in the activities the body wants to do. So there is a mind-body connection which has now been treated with hormones. With molecular biology understanding and at the cellular level. We have to accept that it is not only the science, and the IVF is not the answer. Otherwise IVF should have given us 100% result in terms of pregnancy. So friends we have discussed all the levels and then to surrender and keep the mind open and it becomes an easy conception, pregnancy and delivery. After putting the ova and semen in Petri dish and trying to make sperm enter the ova and its failure, so zona pelicida was dissected and sperm was put inside the ova, then also the conception did not occur.

So these are various procedures that are made in IVF. But we have already discussed the factors which brings about the failure. So this is about the success rate of IVF and failure.

Now we have studied that anatomical and physiological axis, we have considered the psychological factors and the causes of infertility and its solutions. We have studied about the ovulation as well as negative and positive post-coital test.

PCOD—Polycystic Ovarian Disease is becoming very common. At all the ages; right from the time of 13-14 from the time of adolescence to menopausal and post-menopausal women suffer from PCOD. The explanations are many, the drugs are many. The latest is that you put stem cells on the thickened wall of the ovary and it might help. Yes, all thess causes can be handled but to the surprise of our treatment, the ladies came and said that we are having PCOD and we cannot conceive and after explaining the axis of anatomy, physiology, and giving indirect and direct hypnosis, we have succeeded in bringing about pregnancy and taking to full term. So, I want to tell you that belief system is a very important fact in life in so many psychosomatic conditions. When the person is sure that it's not going to happen but unconscious has sorted out the reservations and to their surprise it has happened. The patients came to us when they missed their period, to say to just confirm whether they are pregnant or not, because pregnancy test came back positive. On ultrasound at 6 weeks when we show them the heart pulsating, they are very very happy and so many times we saw that we had to take them through 9 months and later on after delivery to get accustomed to have a child on the breast and after an year they came, bringing the baby who is 1 year old. So this is life and this is the story of a couple wanting to be parents and we are trying to help them with the psychological block, their belief system and acceptance to become the parent.

Thank you very much for patient listening. All the best to the couple. Thank you.

The following are some of the scripts used. They can be delivered in order or separately depending upon the need of the subject. Names have been abbreviated/changed to maintain anonymity.

1.

Dr. Bhaskar Vyas:

"We will like to let you know that Rajni & I, we have been in a hardcore medical profession. She, as you know is one of the senior most gynaecologist in India while I am one of the senior most plastic surgeons in India. We have done our speciality work with extension to further studies in consciousness.

Consciousness is commonly known that either we are conscious or we may be asleep and if we are asleep, then also some people can answer yes and no. Most of the times all of us have had dreams also. We have dreamt various kinds of dreams.

Apart from these 3 states of consciousness, we are now here to introduce you to a 4th stage. The 4th stage of consciousness is classically described in various Indian ancient scripts. The 4th state in Sanskrit is known as *Turya*. This was not known to the West till a couple of centuries ago. Now the West also has woken up to this 4th state and intense scientific studies are on in Europe including England, and America. While England, Europe and USA have recognized this 4th state as a hypnotherapeutic state, India which has really known and generated this knowledge, we are still groping in the dark. There are very few hypnotherapists in India. So, that is the reason why we have to talk across so many miles with the help of such contraptions. But we will salute that kind of scientist; let us salute that kind of scientist who has made us to meet on Zoom or now meeting on Google. Where were these scientists when they thought of discovering this kind of contraptions? Let us pause... pause and think... yes. When SB has nodded his head, i know that he has liked the question.

There was a scientist called Steve Jobs. Steve Jobs wandered in the Himalayas and got that kind of vibrations that has put this kind of facilities in our hand that we are able, not only to listen and talk to each other, but I am seeing some expression on the face of Dr. AB as well.

Now, Dr. AB, I like to tell you, this state of wonder, this state of excitement... this state of excitement, and a sudden discovery of an 'Aha!' experience. You have, both of you have worked on difficult situations, from a business point of view, from a professional point of view and when we steer around a very difficult corner, maybe while driving the car. That time also, for a fraction of a second, 'Oh! I made it. How nice! I made it'. And a difficult situation getting resolved in a flicker of a moment, that also happens and then all of us have had 'Aha!' experience. Now, one wonderful 'Aha!' experience that Dr. AB probably has missed and I would like to be wrong, but my assumption is based on certain solid facts. One 'Aha!' experience is the delivery of a baby. Dr. AB is still to have that 'Aha!' experience that comes when a woman for the first time experiences, 'Oh. My baby! My baby is crying' and the moment she has the baby, the newly born mother, I would say a woman who was a mother to be, but always wanted to be and has not experienced motherhood so far, the first cry of my baby... my baby... my child... my soul... part of my part... body of my body and soul of my soul... my creation. That is a 'Aha!' experience which is a natural due to each and every female in any species and most specifically a human female that is a woman. And subsequently there are 'Aha!' experiences to come. The first touch of the infant baby on the breast, that is engorged with the milk now. And the soft tender lips of the baby, as they start strongly sucking on to the engorged nipple. Yes, I give you milk that is the soul of my soul that will nourish you... that will nourish you not only with galactose and various other food constituents but the most precious constituent that as a mother I give to my child... my baby... is my love.

Take a deep deep breathe Dr. AB and take a deep breath SB. Take a deep deep breath and both of you relax. Wherever you are, it is your natural due now to start the experience of the 4th state and as you listen to my voice, you are listening to my voice and with so much of concern for such wonderful people, so highly educated, so sensible about their situation in life, so discerning to be able to make a definite choice... a discerning choice... you have made a discerning and well informed choice that both of you have decided to be parents now. Take a deep... deep breath. Deeper and deeper still and as you take a deeper breath, you find that your eyes are... your eyes are feeling... eyes are getting blurred and your eyelids are getting heavier and heavier and heavier so that you are finding... you are finding difficulty to keep the eyes open. Your eyelids are heavier and as they are so heavy as if they are like made up of lead. The lead curtains are so heavy that they close by themselves. As you close your eyes or as your eyes have closed, so spontaneously... your eyes are now turning inwards and what is happening all over the cerebral cortex that is well within the skull or what is happening... what is happening in the deep recesses of your heart. The heart is pulsating something like 70 beats per minute and as you see your heart slowing down, at long last... at long last my heart has found a corner... a corner within my body where there is peace. Let there be peace, let there be harmony. Let there be harmony between two lovely individuals whom nature has brought together as two partners. Two partners that have decided to pay back to the humanity what humanity has to be propagated with... Deep... Deep breath... and deeper breath still... And as you breathe deeper and deeper but slower the heart rate beats and there is a feeling of relaxation all over the body. AB has so relaxed... AB has relaxed so that... how would AB like to relax and what does the relaxation indicate? All these questions are forgotten... All these questions are forgotten... "

Dr. Rajni Vyas:

> "Very nice AB. You have put your head on the table but you are listening to what we are talking to you and enjoy this relaxation for a while which relaxes your whole body from head to toe, from front to back and wonderful feeling. Joyful, happy experience for a while till there are a few moments of quietness all around you. Yes AB and SB... both of you are enjoying and make yourself comfortable by taking deep breath. Yes SB very nice. This is a comfortable position. Both of you are feeling relaxed when... "

Dr. Bhaskar Vyas:

> "Dr. Vyas is now taking over once again and I would like to tell you... I am telling you now that relaxation is like what happens, what happens to the soil. The soil that is inundated... inundated with very incessant rain.. the incessant rain that is pouring on even the

hard of the hardest soil, finally the earth, it is natural due of the earth to have the rain. Now that there is a raining of the molecules, when AB and SB are in their own private corner in their own bedroom and there is so much of flow of reciprocal love, SB is pouring so much of tender... tender, loving care and as AB's lips... AB's lips are feeling the wetness... AB's lips are wet with the saliva and AB may want to wet her lips a little more... let your tongue wet your lips AB and as you do so, that wetness, that softness, that is relaxation. As the tender loving care is being poured on several parts of AB 's personal self, AB feels... AB feels tender loving care of the hand... SB has his hands on AB's breast and there is such pleasant tightness in AB's nipples that is relaxation. That tightness that SB would have and is experiencing. SB is experiencing the same tightness as it is in the nipples of AB's breast in SB's penis is also so tight and so erect and how wonderful. This is the organ of creation that the nature has bestowed upon us and it is an organ that is bestowed with a subtle pleasure. The pleasant pleasure that no other organ has. The pleasure pleasantness... pleasantness and the pleasure... as some hands are caressing on the inner side of the thighs... inner sides of the thighs of AB and AB now knows... AB now knows what that relaxation is and when the relaxation... the rain has now continued to pour as a pleasant drizzle. There is such pleasant drizzle and that is relaxation. That has made... the rain makes the soil wet and such a rain sometimes, SB is so anxious to pour in that it may just spurt out. Never mind. Never mind SB. This, with your virility, with your vigour, with your youthfulness, you can do it again and again. Let now AB pour love. AB is pouring love on to the lips of SB and such tender loving care, such gentleness, such playing about the penis. Both of you are made for each other. AB and SB are made for each other. The nature is vibrating the song of the song that AB and SB are made for each other and when such suppleness, such softness, such tenderness, loving care, AB feels the wetness, the softness, all over her vagina. It is so soft, so supple, so tender... tender like a petal. Like a flower petal that has opened out. Its opening of a flower that is felt all over inside the vagina and in this subtle and sublime moment of union... subtle and sublime bondage of male and female organs... their consciousness is also united as one. The consciousness of Lord Shiva... Call him Lord Shiva or call him the Eternal, Eminent, Supremely Sublime, Creative Power is now united into the manifestation that will soon emerge... The sperms are in pursuit of an ovum and on the fourteenth day after beginning of the menstruation, once again on 12th, 13th, 14th and 15th day after menstruation, SB and AB will listen to this recorded cassette on all these four consecutive days in their private, peaceful place. They will make love and there will be an ovum... there will be an ovum that will receive a sperm and a baby will be created. This is not only a promise from Dr. Rajni Vyas, Dr. Bhaskar Vyas, we are duty-bound to make this promise because you are such wonderful people and what is ordinarily awarded, even to the most menial of human beings, how could nature deny such a gift to such wonderful people. The promise is from your friend like Rajni and Bhaskar, but it is also the promise of Mother nature and mother nature awards whatever is the natural due to each and every one regardless of whatever reservations... where are the reservations now? The reservations are gone, we are united together in this private corner of our life. We are privileged that AB and SB have shared this personal private experience which is our indeed a great privilege. We are also feeling blessed that we are some way helpful to you in the pursuit of your most natural and great creation. Listen to this cassette once again on 12th, 13th, 14th and 15th day of menstrual cycle and after listening to the cassette, make love and you will create a wonderful baby."

Dr. Rajni Vyas:

"Yes AB and SB, you have experienced this wonderful experience by Dr. Vyas and both of you have cooperated, enjoyed and continue to relax till you are happy, convinced that both of you are made for each other. And wanting to go ahead and are creating a newcomer in your life and when there is full convincing situation, you will gradually, quietly wake up, take your own time... take your own time to wake up and after your means when you wake up... Yes, AB, you have woken up. Fine. Alert. Stretch your arms... stretch your arms in front of you... move from side to side... yes AB, you have woken up well. And maybe after your meals you may go to sleep again. Get fully awake. And SB, take your own time to wake up... but it is the time to wake up for your meals... and SB as I count for you 10 to 1... Yes, as I am counting and you are listening and it is 10... and 9... SB you are listening to me... 10 to 9 and to 8... very good, very nice... SB move side to side, from stretched hands, move your neck with the hand and you are alert. Nice... very nice... yes. If you have a glass of water by your side, just sip it. Very nice... and as you will be swallowing you will feel the relaxation... as you are swallowing you will feel alert, relaxed and happy... You have done a wonderful job and I am very happy. Both of us want to congratulate you for experiencing this relaxation... Yes SB, wake up... maybe have another sip of water both of you... Very nice... take your own time to wake up and if you have any question to ask or just want to be that is fine... SB you may not drive now soon. After an hour or so you may drive... have your meals or have some bite...

Actually we wanted both of you to be together to have lunch... We have really succeeded in making this long distance... though so near... this agenda to work out and both of us are congratulating you and wake up... "

2.

We have already made friends... sometimes the situation so arises that people make instantaneous friendship... what I would call in a jiffy! Jiffy is so small a time, and yet in a small time... one or two and one such three people... such three people also make such good friends that they start understanding the language of the heart... the language of the heart is the language that heart speaks and heart receives... who has already been in a good relationship... in a relationship that would have gone to intense friendship... intense friendship or let us say... let us say in a relationship of love... in such a relationship, in love, there is no... there is no... there is no business of buy and sell... there is no accounting as to who has given what... and that kind of a relationship where giving is much more pleasurable... I repeat, giving is much more pleasurable but then the recipient has kept no account whatsoever... giving is so much more... giving is so much more joy but when the recipient has not kept any account whatsoever, how can we calculate that would be only futile... this kind of a relationship between you two partners have promised and before putting into verbal or any kind of love letter... or any kind of document, you have already exchanged... this experience may amount... the experience without your understanding about hypnosis or without even knowing what hypnosis is, you have already... you may have already exchanged... I trust this kind of noble... this kind of noble relationship is what I meant by the word divine in the previous session... where there is no trade, there is no commerce, there is so much of joy in giving and the receiving is not accountable... so taking a review of what you might have already experienced... or what you might be waiting to happen. I am inclined for a small revision; the revision begins with:

Q. 1: Did you find yourself into... in a different state than what is ordinarily awake sleep and dream during last two sessions?

Q. 2: The last two sessions, each one of them, with your estimation of time would have lasted for how long?

Q. 3: Whether you experienced a sense of well being... a sense of euphoria? for those who are not familiar I define Euphoria as a sense of great joy.

Q. 4: Did you feel any kind of smell... your most favorite smell that ordinarily was not in the room where you listened... where you listened to our session?

Next question: Did you see multiple Red Roses in a... red roses in a Rose garden?

Next question: Did you see a whole panorama... a whole panorama of various patterns... various patterns of flower beds... various patterns of the flower beds that were made of violet, indigo, blue... violet Indigo blue yellow orange and once again red... but when all 7 colours mix together... they constitute... take a deep breath... and a deeper breath still... let your body relax... and when you see the perfect blend in right proportions, you are seeing the perfect blending of all the colours and they constitute a white... a white... a white flower bed of white roses... White Roses are also so much more beautiful... you cannot think whether to vote for a white rose or whether to choose other kind of coloured rose... and why try to dissect and to analyze... why try to dissect and analyze what is beautiful... beauty is beautiful... beauty is beautiful and so is a love relationship... a love relationship also is beautiful and yet... and yet... we decide most of the things... most of the situations... both of you partners are highly intelligent people... people have made their careers already brilliant, shiningly successful and the pursuit... pursuit of excellence, pursuit of excellence has no limits... to such people what is their natural due would have already accrued and they have already... they have already experienced the trance but may also... may also be in a deeper trance... however *Turya*... however *Turya* is a natural due of the entire mankind it is known that different people have different levels of hypnotizability... let us say most successful people would have been intelligent and when they would have pursued... when they would have limited their pursuit into a very well focalized beam... a very well focalized beam, that would have generated such a brilliant successful career... in the process, they would have put aside several other things... several other things that they could have naturally... naturally... and I keep on repeating the word 'Naturally'... they would have naturally achieved... so, in case your experience tells you that you would like to... you would like to have a deeper experience... like to have a deeper experience of *Turya*, the naturally occurring 4th state of consciousness, it is once again your natural due and by giving you additional inputs, we... we are going... we are going to gain both ways... those who have experienced only a slight dream-like state would find further ways... refined tools to take their experience deeper... and those who have already experienced deeper states of *Turya* will be able to take it onto a more subtler level... subtler level... I repeat... S. U. B. T. L. E.R... subtler level that can only be experienced when doors of unconscious mind get wide open and with such a revelation, joy abounds... so whatever may be your earlier experience, we... we repeat another experience... and that will be to take *Turya* into deeper and higher modes... So you might think something more elaborate... something more intricate and something really difficult, you might need to do... but, what is natural... what is natural, that flows naturally... and what flows naturally is what nature does... nature has its own... nature has its own way of finding out a flow as almost all rivers... almost all rivers all over the world find... do... and flow... find, do and flow... so, let us go to even more easier way and a natural way as a first exercise... first exercise to deepen hypnosis...

Now you know and I do not have to elaborate that the body... entire body is almost closed by skeletal muscles... there are muscles maybe thin in the forehead, but try to wrinkle your forehead... yes, you can do it... try to give a smile, and you can do it so easily... try to move your head to and fro... and so natural... All this happens because the muscles contract and relax... let us just do only 1 thing... that 1 thing is relaxation... R.E.L.A.X.A.T.I.O.N... relaxation... relax all the toe muscles... all muscles of your 10 toes and when you can relax, wriggle your toes... wriggle your toes and throw all the tension from your body... those 10 toes are in their natural state of relaxation... and see and feel how different they are to what they were before... and having known this, you relax all the muscles of both your ankles... your both ankles are now relaxed and they feel so much easy and feel so much good... so why not extend this feeling so that the long muscles that surround your ankle... they are also relaxed... and relax the muscles of the left... relax the muscles surrounding the left ankle... and find that it is natural for the right sided muscle to follow your command... to follow your command to relax not only the long muscles of your leg but also the other muscles... surrounding your right knee... right thigh... relax them... R.E.L.A.X... relax the left sided muscles of your knee and thigh... how wonderful... how wonderful it is to see that the other muscles of the left sided knee and thigh have also relaxed... feel the fountain... feel the fountain of relaxation springing up right from your sole all the way up to not only the thighs, but also the groin.. the fountain flourishes from the groin... from the groin to the back of the spine... and the same time the fountain also... fountain also spreads upwards onto your groin muscles. Your abdominal muscles... goes up and up to the lumbar muscles and let them relax... and this is at your command... they have acquired greater mastery on your muscular system so that they not only contract at your wish... they did it so... but now they will relax as you command them to go up... your neck droops by the side... your jaw may also so relax that it droops and as the relaxation spreads higher, you try not to close your eyes... your eyes are surround by circular muscles and you are trying to keep your eyes open and find how difficult it is to keep them open... when every muscle in your body wants to relax, how impossible it is to keep your eyes open and let your eyelids also close and as your eyelids have closed, you are experiencing a deeper, a subtler and profound peace, tranquillity and joy... Jo chahe wo ho jaye... let every noble wish of your heart be fulfilled... the promises are given... the promises are given and they will be fulfilled.

3.

The power within the mind or the power of the mind... and the mind that is so powerful may have been... I believe you are highly intelligent... profoundly educated and motivated... motivated with a natural wish... natural wish to the entire mankind... natural wish from within the heart so you would have had what all... what all the total kind of relaxation you can experience and that can lead to a deeper, more peaceful state of mind that is something that should be elementary for most intelligent people... however if you wish... only and only if you really wish there are still subtler ways the present day world... particularly highly educated people like you want more obvious, physically visible and repeatable and reproducible... . I repeat... in the scientific world objectivity, demonstrability, reproducibility are the need... these qualities you already possess... and not only 1... there are, I would say we are in a position to physically demonstrate how your mind is so powerful as... so powerful as to bring about quite some strange and not so easily explainable... . I repeat, not so easily explainable... but surely physically demonstrable... more than 1 such method... to suit your sensibility as a highly intelligent person... so that you may want the information in dots... so the three methods that we can still experience and demonstrate are... 1 levitation of the arm... 2. A coin gathering weight... a coin gathering weight from the atmospheric particles... 3 anaesthesia... . I repeat a certain part can be made not to feel any sensation including pain and as a subheading further transfer of the anaesthesia that is loss of all the sensation including... including pain... transfer of anaesthesia... total... total loss of feeling pain sensation that is anaesthesia... from your anaesthetized hand onto another part of your body, say cheek... anaesthesia is the final, ultimate, most powerful demonstration about how... how hypnosis... how does the hypnosis change bring about a paradigm shift so that something most unusual can also happen... however, in order to demonstrate the last, you will have to travel to a hypnotherapist and your physical presence before a hypnotherapist is necessary... we would wish that sensible people, even in a short demonstration of the other two would want to avoid... to avoid going personally to a hypnotherapist... if we have become enough of friends to trust... and because you have trusted, you have listened to all these sessions, invested your valuable time... in search of... in quest of a resolution, what is your natural due... I have repeated, and I shall repeat again and again... what shall be happening as the happening of change of seasons or happening of morning after night that should have happened to you and we know that your systems are alright... Your ovaries are functioning normally, the spermatozoa are being produced by the testes... or if the count is low, if the ovulation is irregular, that is why we term this as unexplained reproductive failure... the explanation in within your mind... the explanation in within your mind... where is the block that the entire hypnosis process. Now at this stage you have started understanding the power of your mind... so let us call the process as hypnoanalysis... hypnoanalysis is as scientific as the psychoanalytic method as initially enunciated by Sigmund Freud... but what Sigmund Freud and his subsequent followers even of today... Freudian method sometimes takes 6 months and even then... even then there is no validation... there is psychoanalytic... psychoanalysis does not provide any validation while now we are going to the next step... next step of a physical demonstration about an objective proof... an objective proof that your mind does work wonders... and one of the wonders is that your mind... your mind only has blocked a natural occurrence of conception and such a natural occurrence... this hindrance can easily be removed by the power of your mind... we have seen that you can relax... re... lax... RELAX... relax... let go all the tensions from the feet, from the muscles of your toes, from the muscles of your sole and let the relaxation spread upwards to the ankle and feel good... so good to feel relaxed... and from the fountain of relaxation springing... springing from the sole of your feet, how cool, pleasant, peaceful it feels to have found this fountain of peace and let it spared upwards...

it has gone up, up and further up so that the muscles around your ankles are relaxed and as they relax, feel calm, cool... calm, cool, composed... you are feeling calm, cool, composed so that your muscles relax further into the calf muscles, into the muscles of all the muscles of the leg... let them relax... the muscles of your legs are relaxed and as the fountain is springing upwards now rapidly, let the thigh muscles... the muscles of your back... the muscles in front of your body are relaxed... let the fountain of relaxation further go into your left arm, your right arm, both the forearms... all the 10 fingers... all the 10 fingers of both the hands... your shoulder muscles are relaxed and your neck is relaxed further and maybe it bends on one of the sides... and by this time you have found that your eyelids have become so heavy... they have become as if they are made from lead sheets... your eyelids are so heavy that they are made up of lead sheets and they are already closed... in this profound, easily enjoyable state something strange has already started happening to your right.,. right shoulder... right elbow... right wrist... right fingers... what kind of strange happening is this?? What is happening to your right hand that it has started becoming lighter, lighter and further lighter than the air... AHA!!... AHAA!! Oh, of course my right hand, you tell yourself, my right hand has become so light that it has started lifting upwards... it goes up right from the place it was resting in your lap or maybe on the chair handle, it has started lifting and as it lifts, it takes wrist along... wrist along... the wrist also has lost weight... and like a feather, your right.

4.

My dear dear friends. My dear dear friends, we have already worked together in collaboration. There is a collaboration that will create something grand, special. Grand and special creation and the process... process is to be executed by... the process is to be executed by you two partners. In this creative process, I am along with Dr. Rajni Vyas, is a facilitator and the facilitation has already begun. The facilitation has already begun when you consented out of your own choice and selection of... out of your own choice to facilitate a natural process. Does a river need facilitation to flow? You are highly intelligent. Very well educated people and yet you pause... may be you have paused to think over... does a river need to be facilitated to flow? Have you had the remembrance of your childhood innocence? I remind you... I remind you... go back in time and see yourself... see yourself playing in a school ground. Maybe playing on a school swing and you know that when you swing on a swing... when you go on a swing, maybe a single person, or along with a friend, the swing... the swing has natural tendency to swing back and forth. A swing has a natural tendency to swing back and forth... That way the seasons also... the seasons round the year also rotate... winter will be followed by spring and the spring will have... the flowers will naturally bloom as spring will naturally... the spring will naturally be followed by summer and summer will be followed... so on and so forth... so on and so forth.

So it is also natural for 98% of the people... I repeat, in our vast experience of over 45 years... in our vast experience of over 45 years, those we do not call them patients. They are not patients but they are special kind of human beings who even challenge... the special kind of human beings who even challenge the natural process of experiencing and you may be... you may be that kind of special human being who have either only marginally or with little depth... but you will want still to experience... you may want to experience even greater and deeper... greater and deeper state of hypnosis. It is your choice and as your eyelids have started becoming already heavy and if you have already feeling difficult... it is difficult to keep your eyes open... you are already on the fast track, but we want to go even faster... and a fast track can be... a fast track is being accelerated with even faster and superfast... superfast train with your eyes almost closed, you are seeing... yes, you are seeing a faster train and the faster train is being replaced... is already replaced with superfast train and you see... you see now even if your eyes have been really half closed, even if your eyelids do not like to remain open, I suggest for a very novel and a special experience you keep your eyes open... How wonderful! How talented! That is what I expected of both of you that... that... that with the expectation of a special, special gift that you are endowed with... very very few people are endowed with this kind of a gift that even when their eyelids want to close, they are able to keep them open. Now that you have kept your eyelids open, you stretch out one of your hands... right from shoulder onto the elbow to the wrist all along at the shoulder level... All along at the shoulder level. Your preferred hand is stretched out and you have put... you have put a coin... may be a coin that may be like one rupee coin. It doesn't matter what mint... it doesn't matter what mint, and what year the coin is printed. We know that the coins printed in different years do... the coins though of same denomination may and do weigh... they do weigh slightly differently... this is commonly known that a rupee coin that you are holding no... you are now holding in a difficult to keep open eyes but you are able to keep them open and you are seeing the coin in your palm... palm that is being held in your outstretched hand... never mind that you are finding it difficult to keep the eyes open because I want and you will surely experience what I want that... I want you to be aware of a special faculty... the power that now you will see... a power that is always there and yet it is so common that you require... you require this special perceptive state... a special perceptive state that you are in now... The power has already been there... it was there before, but now you will experience that the coin in the palm of your hand... the coin in the palm of your hand is constantly, all the time being bombarded. The coin is being bombarded by very very small... very very small particles from the atmosphere. This was known only to select, specially perceptive, *Rishis*... and now your perception is as powerful... as powerful as to the first *Rishi*... the first *Rishi* who had experienced, who had even seen those very small... very very minutely small... minutely small, ordinarily not visible particles that now... that now the coin in your hand is receiving from the atmosphere and again... highly educated and highly intelligent persons that you are, you know that howsoever a particle... a particle is a particle is a particle because it certainly has... a particle has some weight. A particle has some weight. Some particles have been constantly bombarding themselves onto the coin... onto the coin... The particles have been bombarding onto the coin in the palm of your hand and even a small particle has some weight. So, you are now capable of sensing... sensing what you have not been ordinarily giving a pass. That smallest particle has weight and so, what a miracle! What a miracle that the weight... the weight of the coin has started increasing. This may appear to be a miracle but your special power to perceive even the smallest difference now has made this seemingly miracle like occurrence happen. Aha! How nice. How wonderful to have this special power to see a happening that the weight... weight of... weight of the coin in your hand... in the palm of your hand has increased. Now it goes on increasing. Increasing... and increasing at every moment. At every moment, thousands of small, minute particles from the atmosphere are being deposited onto the palm... onto the coin... onto the coin in the palm of your hand and the weight... the weight of the coin... the weight... the weight of the coin is increasing. It is increasing maybe... yes surely now by leaps and bounds and as the weight of the coin is increasing, even your powerful hand has started... Your powerful hand... Your powerful hand that is holding the coin has started shaking. Naturally. When the weight of the coin has increased, even the powerful hand can only hold... a powerful hand can only hold up to a limit. A weight that is within its natural power and see with your open eyes that .. see with your open eyes that are really difficult to hold that your powerful hand is now trembling. The powerful hand is now trembling. Who is moving... who is moving your palm? Who makes your palm and forearm tremble? And what is making your shoulder also to shake?

As you are now able to... you are now able to actually witness what Rishi Kanaad... Yes... There was once before a time, there was a Rishi who was able to see this minute, tiniest most particles that have constantly bombarded the coin in your palm. That is why he was called Rishi Ka-Naad: 'Kanaad'. I repeat, Rishi was called, Rishi Ka-naad. Yes you will want to know the spelling so I give you the spelling for his name. It is K for King, A for Alfred, N for New York, A again for Alfred and D. Ka-Naad. D for a donkey.

And now seeing... seeing a virtual image of Kanaad Rishi within your archetypal memory... archetypal memory that goes back even to thousands of years back you find... you find that the coin... the coin has shaken... is shaking so very much in the palm of your hand that you are not able... you are not able to hold it... you are not able to hold it in the palm of your hand and... and... and... the coin drops on the ground. The coin drops on the ground. Your outstretched hand at the shoulder also drops into your left... Your eyes have spontaneously closed. Aha! What relaxation! What peace! What tranquillity!

A river howsoever turbulent during the floods... howsoever turbulent during Russian revolution... once there is peace and tranquillity, even the quiet flows the don. Feel at peace. Tranquillity... Calm, cool, composed, with closed eyes. Be absolutely sure that when nature is allowed its own ways, it flows quietly, naturally as much surely as D.A.W.N. follows the night. So would your physiology, your various hormonal cycles in the body will flow naturally as much as the phases of the moon. It is indeed as great privilege... great privilege for Dr. Rajni and me, that is Bhaskar Vyas that we have had... we have had your trust and confidence in this collaboration. The promises are given and they will be surely fulfilled.

Thank you.

5. Male-Azoospermia to Normal Count Stress

Friends. Having worked with you in collaborative mode in the process of procreating. Procreating a new creation. Entirely a creation such as that was never there before and would never be duplicated entirely... Yes. It is indeed a great privilege for us that now I consider... I consider that I have earned myself... I have earned myself to address... to address you two special persons in quest... in search of creativity. And what a creativity search you have engaged yourself in. A search of creativity... A search and a surge... s.u.r.g.e. surge of creativity is already in process so that son enough you will be rewarded. You will be rewarded surely and certainly... You will be rewarded with a baby. Running so fast... Yes, you have been excellent students. Always in search of excellence and then excelling in your professional work. You have risen from one peak... . one peak to another... Such excellent people can so excel that they certainly and surely have succeeded in each and every aim. Whatever milestone you have set for yourself... Whatever milestone that you have set for yourself, you have achieved... Surely and certainly. You have right in your high school days, understood the process of reproduction... Take a deep breath... A further deep, deep and deeper breath and... feel the process of hypnosis creeping slowly, certainly... Right from the bottom... bottom that is the sole of your feet. You are now feeling relaxed in the sole of the feet and a fountain of relaxation is creeping over... is springing like a fountain... like a fountain, it is creeping upwards from the sole of the feet. Onto your legs, onto your knees, onto your thighs... And you have done this before. So easy for you to do it again, so that finally it is fast moving upwards. Upwards onto your thighs, onto you loin... In front of the abdomen as well as on to the back... back of your spine and it moves far forward, upwards so that both your shoulders are so relaxed that they have drooped. The relaxed shoulders drooped down by themselves. And in this relaxation process, you have hardly realized that your eyelids are so relaxed that they have closed by themselves. And yet, we are connected... for friends to connect with each other is so easy. But, having established through a special medium of hypnosis, we are established through a special connection of hypnosis. That is connecting in consciousness... Connecting in consciousness of a different kind where heart speaks, and heart listens and heart follows and whatever has been desired, happens... *Jo Maange, Wo Ho Jaye...* and these two creative hearts are desiring and definitely deserving to be rewarded with a child. So, *Jo Maange, Wo Ho Jaye*, this process of hypnotherapy is a medium where the currency... the happening is that what is intensely wished for as a natural process... natural process of creation is something that happens spontaneously and you have such powerful minds that your powerful lifestyle... your pursuit of excellence... your pursuit of excellence has even blocked a natural process of reproduction. And now I wish to focus on the factors that would have contributed through the male partner.

My dear friend... Muscularity is coupled with responsibility. Generally, in reproductive failure, here it usually happens that women go the investigations first and when their tests show that they are functioning normally... their menstrual cycle is normal... even their ovulation occurs between 12 to 14th day of the menstrual cycle. Then, the male does get his... the male does get his semen examined. Herein lies a substantial evidence as to how... a substantial evidence to show as to how mind dominates the physiological processes as well. Let us go step by step as to what... what factors through the medium of mind could have dominated the physiological process. We are not talking about some of the very strange and curious and yet very very few instances where we have come across mature, successful, young people thinking that they are having a normal intercourse. We must exclude... we must exclude such couples because when they had not undergone the notional understanding... Elementary facts that an intercourse is as simple as a piston... sexual intercourse is as simple as a piston fitting into a barrel... Maybe its a surprise... and it should be a surprise to you because you are far more intelligent than not to understand as to how... how a syringe and the piston fits with each other. And by the very definition, such ignorant people do not account for the couples like yours... highly intelligent... highly educated and having normal sexual intercourse... that kind of people we are addressing here. And in the sexual act, the responsibility is to initiate the act by the male. Most of the time, the sex act is initiated by the male... It is also seen that the partners who have come across each other and marred out of love... married out of love as a love marriage... even surmounting the obstacles that orthodox caste system, social restrictions and so on when it comes to sharing the bed... Two loving, caring for each other, capable of taking responsibilities of high paid successful jobs... the male finds... the male partner finds that he is dominated by his loved one... that can result in what a surprise of surprise... that can result in failure of erection of penis and on the other hand, too much of excitement would have caused him to have premature ejection... premature ejection causes him to have a failure of penetration once again... If this is the case... if this is the case, there is plenty of time in one night. There is plenty of time, not to be disappointed at all... continue to caress each other... continue to excite the female partner. The lady who is already aroused in her sexuality should deploy several ways gentle, caressing and certainly with patience so that after a short while the man... the dominant partner in the sex act... the partner responsible... the male partner. The dominant one, once again rediscovers his dominant role and is able to penetrate the penis into the vagina and so as to have a second ejaculation... But, it can so happen that the woman partner... the lady has excelled far, far, far beyond in external profession career. So that, times and again in the family life, in the friend circle, in the social life, the man has to play the second fiddle. Our society is so oriented that... our society is oriented to the male dominance and a husband or maybe all husbands are still to be accustomed to the term as househusbands. The word housewife may be found in a dictionary. But in a psychology profile of most gender of humankind male have not... have not a psychological profile of househusband. Here, the therapy is focused on the fact that ego strengthening of the male can easily be achieved that in the usual posture of sexual act... usual posture of sexual act is performed... is performed... usual performance of sexual act is done with the man mounting on the female. It is the male who mounts the female. It is the penis that penetrates the vagina and against one ovum, man has capacity to ejaculate millions of sperms at one time.

We now look at a paradoxical situation whereby the sperm examination... examination of spermatic fluid in a pathology lab reveals that there are very few sperms or there is no sperms at all... that is termed as azoospermia. The doctor has erroneously proclaimed since there are no sperms, there will be no baby. Profoundly incorrect, dear, dear doctor friend. You have not taken the correct history of the environment in which the family is living. There could have been very tragic... so tragic as to be having numerous deaths in the near and dear friends in the family and if that is the case, mind certainly recovers from this post traumatic stress syndrome. Time is the best healer and this trauma may be by itself, or with this kind of hypnotherapy sessions, will also be healed. There is another observations that we have frequently come across in our practice. That is a common occurrence for the investors in the stock market. Stock market is known to have radical ups and downs. And at every dip, some investors are suddenly left with large losses. With a large loss in the stock market, a large loser is also prone as it has frequently been noted in our practice, to have oligospermia, that is sudden decrease in the sperm count or even azoospermia. A wise and experienced investor knows the stock market and its undulations. He must assure himself that like the stock market, his sperm count will also bounce back once the environment of happiness, joy, pleasure and ease pervades.

So, brace up your shoulders my dear responsible male partner. Nature has given you the prerogative of being predominant. The society and the social metrics has made our society male oriented, male dominant society and so has the nature made you a predominant performer in the sexual act. It would be but natural for you to act naturally and live up to your responsibility and surely Mother Nature will reward both of you with a baby. There is no need to hurry to adopt a child. We have come across several instances where couples with unexplained reproductive failure gave up hope and adopted a baby. Once the anxiety, worries, so many disappointments at failure in assisted reproductive failure... reproductive failures that occur following several attempts at assisted reproduction with a test tube baby and so on. When a baby was adopted, the worry, anxiety, unnecessary expense and repeated disappointments were gone. The couple have got success in having a baby. So let there be no hurry. You will also succeed and be rewarded in a natural course, naturally.

We are indeed happy. Dr. Rajni and I, Bhaskar Vyas are indeed very privileged to have collaborated with you in this noble of the noblest task of creating a new human being.

Thank you

6.

We have understood about Alice being in Wonderland. We have also seen the situation about not only Alice herself and a friend of Alice... Both have experienced... Both of them have experienced what it is to be in the Wonderland that is Hypnosis as experience... Now some people and probably the most of highly intelligent people as both of you are... have various depths of hypnotherapy. The hypnotherapeutic work does progress... the work does get done... either a person experience light hypnosis or medium or deep trance... this will surely happen, though deeper the hypnosis more inner depth experience goes all the way... all the way... deep down in the innermost layer of deep unconscious mind... since you have... you have been highly intelligent, and highly intelligent people already know the three different levels of depths where a suggestion or a suggestion that may entirely... may entirely be understood in a different context... afterall words are meant to convey what they mean... but when in a state of hypnosis, the words do take a altogether different meaning... and that meaning is more likely to convey the innermost, hidden, something that has been suppressed, that has been constantly trying to express in the outer sense and yet is usually not understood even when clearly paraphrased... But... but what was not understood for so many many days, many many months, maybe many years, suddenly reveals what, where, how, why something... Something that is a natural due... natural due is... natural due is naturally bestowed by Nature... Nature has created... nature has created obviously 2 distinctly different sexes. This is clear and obvious all across the human race that there are 2 human... 2 human variants... in every species, each and every species creates a male and a female and even a child understands that there are... there are girls and there are boys and together... together and together only it is the girls and the boys... the women and the men... together they move the entire world... having understood this elementary truth, let us first review what... let us first review what you may have experienced through the previous session... I would like that you review that whether you have experienced the

4th state... the 4th state of consciousness that we call... we call as Hypnosis but hypnosis is something that we all have known without understanding or only with a glimpse... just a glimpse and have not thought much about it... so, when you have had a 1st time experience of hypnotherapy, look within... look, look within... let your eyes look within, into the depth of your heart, into various, various levels of *Turya* experience and... and grade your experience of hypnosis into light, medium and deep... Deep hypnotherapeutic experience even after you are made to come out... even after you have started doing your regular work, or maybe you may have gone to sleep for some time, regardless hypnotherapeutic work does go on... that happens even in medium trance as well as in superficial trance... however, you feel you had no fundamental change... no fundamental change in your level of consciousness in *Turya* please mark it down and we shall apply several strategies... there are numerous strategies available... do not and do not... do not despair... do not give up... What is your natural due and every man... every man it is said, a child is the father of man... do you agree? A child is the father of a man... and every mother... every girl child is born as a girl child so as she may... every girl has a natural right... each and every girl does have a natural right to motherhood... she... that is every woman... every woman is destined to be a creator... she creates and eventually having conceived, nurtured carefully for 3 months, 6 months, 9 months... at the right time... she gives... Mother Nature gives a fully grown... Mother Nature gives back what every mother is naturally has a right to have... We have numerous examples... more than 550 couples... 550 couples having unexplained reproductive failure. They had a good sperm count, women had normally occurring ovulation between 13th to 15th day of menstruation... and so on... and why should such a couple... why should such a couple not have a baby?... that the experts have been able... the experts without further investigation whatever you have already understood and already got established that the spermatogenesis and the ovulation are occurring normally, then what is the obstacle? That is the reason why you have sought our help and we are duty bound... we are duty bound that we share... we surely impart... not only knowledge for the sake of knowledge but towards the achievement of the ultimate goal for which we are working together now—so having assured you deep in our hearts that we surely understand... we will further explain when we understand... before start of the 3rd session by confirming that you have experienced hypnosis... when you have experienced a finely refined perfume that is a good enough test... and have you not had this kind of experience... we have available two different objective evidence... I repeat, objective appearance, they are not only appearance, but they are visible evidences to prove that you have undergone trance... trance... I repeat... trance is a different state of consciousness... it is your natural right to experience it... to have a deep experience every time you have... every time you have had sex with your partner, and everytime you experience this trance, it is natural... it is nature's given gift... an opportunity to create a new... a new... a new human baby... Let us write down what you experienced and what you have yet to experience and with a review of what we have gained, we shall take the session further...

It is our privilege... it is our privilege of course to be a part of witness... witnessing a creation of a new human baby is a great privilege for us and for that we shall continue our genuine devotional help in the next session... thank you...

7.

The following uses the 'Visit to a garden' suggestions and builds upon it for unexplained reproductive failure

At a visit to the garden. You have been listening few sessions and have leanrt to go into self hypnosis. So please stay comfortably, at peace and start taking deep breath, in and out. I'm sure now you have become experts in going into trance. So as you take a deep breath in, the oxygenated, pure energized air goes into your nostril to the back of the pharynx into trachea, broncha and last to the alveoli and exchanges with carbon dioxide, unwanted chemicals, unwanted thoughts and very very positive approach to anything that you want to do. Even in your routine work that you have found that you are becoming more efficient but at the same time, feel comfortable and creative. You are also surprised with your abilities and this breathing is continuing right from the time of birth and makes the blood absolutely pure, red and starts circulating into the small muscles of your sole and you feel very relaxed in your sole.

Make yourself comfortable, if you want to move and make your position, please make it. And that relaxation moves upwards on the back of your ankle. Move your toes to throw away all the stress, tension, thoughts and let this circulation spread from back of the foot to the front of the foot to the ankle and up. You feel relaxed. And up into the gastrocnemius muscle of the legs and into the knee and this moves fast forward into your thighs. This you have been doing every day and now it goes into the knee, up into the thighs. The big muscles of the thighs and into the abdomen. And all that organs that are there in that Pandora box is completely relaxed and looking bright and it goes into the chest and into both the lungs and heart. And you are listening your heart and breathing deep in and out. Experiencing this relaxation is going to be quiet, comfortable and enjoy this for a few seconds till my voice also goes away.

Yes, very nice. I am back to make you relaxed. Both the shoulders, your forearms, your fingers, and you can move your fingers and make yourself comfortable. Completely quiet and from the neck it goes to the face's small muscles and they relax and you look 10 years younger with that beautiful smile. Yes. Very happy and just keep on taking deep breaths in and out till I come back again. And enjoying this relaxation, the wave goes into your brain and its crevices. Fresh blood is flowing and makes you feel quiet, tranquil and you are in a very comfortable situation. As we are in a very happy mode, and it is cool, early morning, quiet within.

Let us visit the garden. We come in front of the garden. There's a majestic, tall entrance made of steel with a nice design and there are circular steel plates attached which is having so many kinds of figures. You try to watch and gradually enter into the nicely clean path that has been made and on either side there are tall trees. You are listening the birds, the adult birds and the small birds. Various singing notes that they are communicating with which you are appreciating and you are gradually moving forward. The adult birds are ready to fly away and fine breeze touches your cheeks. You hold each other's hand and move up and down feeling that fineness of the breeze. There are small flower beds in between the tall trees of various colours, various fragrances, and of various age. They are small glands and little bigger and little bigger that all this colour and fragrance attracts you, and both of you, hand in hand moving forward enjoying each and every bit of situations and using all your five senses, you walk forward and there is a huge open space which is a nice green colour grass knoll. You put your feet on that ground and want to remove your shoes and chappals because you have seen small dewdrops on that grass. You both remove your shoes and put your feet on the grass and you feel so nice. Pull and want to walk forward and both of you walking hand in hand, walking forwards and from a distance you listen sounds. Musical notes, some laughing loudly, the children's voice and you move forward and you come near a bunch of small children with their guardian and teachers and you stand at a distance and watch them. All those children with the toddlers, to the five to six years with beautiful dresses of various colours. Dark and light, with various designs on that cloth. Nicely combed hair with pink and red ribbons with the girls and boys; well combed hair, some have long and some have short hair and you just stand there, looking at each other, smiling and as if telling that what a nice decision you took today morning to come to this beautiful garden and watching these small children laughing, giggling with their lunchbox in the hand, eating, spilling, running, trying to catch each other and you just try to find out a bench where you can sit and comfortably watch them playing. And as you are watching, you feel so joyful, so happy and suddenly you remember that you have a camera. He gets up and goes near the elder person, the teacher and requests to take a few photographs. And the teacher happily and pleasantly says please go ahead. You start your video, taking round form teacher to teach and the children playing, running and moving around and you stand still but your camera keeps on moving. With a nice background of beautiful blue sky, tall trees, green lawn. Everything is coming in your video and a small toddler you see coming nearer you and you focus on that small toddler who is walking with all the two feet and two hands and you stop the video and start photographing with various position by moving yourself from left to right and going forward and backward and you are so happy that all his moods you have locked into your photographs. And again you go back and sit down on that bench where your partner is sitting and she has also watched it carefully and says thank you for locking them into your heart and into your camera. They are having a picnic and they are sitting down in a circle and have brought some food with them which you also have brought. You eat what these small children being served and eating and there the sunrise occurs and there is so much of bright red light. The sun starts throwing its energy and you feel so happy, satisfied, feeling all this joy in your mind. In your heart. And you decide to go back home. Sitting on your scooter, you gradually drive slowly singing your favourite song. There is hardly any traffic. You are very joyful in your heart and arrive at your home. As he is parking the scooter, you take out the key from your purse and try to open the gate. And there stands your gynaecologist and you are surprised to see her and she takes the key from you and open the doors for you, wide open and you enter and at the back he also enters.

Gynaecologist just disappears and you straight go into your bedroom. The air is so cool and comfortable that you had experienced in the garden. So you open out your windows and draw on the curtains. Both feeling extremely happy watching the toddler's photos hand in hand, you sit down and keep on watching this toddler and have a nice image in your heart.

Smiling face makes you happy looking at each other. You want to have sex and start holding each other's hand, kissing each other. Feeling very happy, relaxed, holding each other lying in your bed. You are having, absolutely happily enjoying the sex. The semen is deposited in the vagina in the cervix and so many sperms run through the external os into the internal os into the endometrium canal and they are in the mouth of the opening of the tube and into the tube and it is the 13th day when the ovulation has occurred and the fimbrial end has picked up the ova that is being liberated by the mature ovum and by movement of the tube, the peristalsis it moves forward and from so many sperms, one dominant sperm enters as other sperms have liquefied and make the surrounding, the lining of the tube very very receptive. Just visualize and enjoy the entering of that sperm into the ovum and conception is occurring.

Blessings from everywhere pour in onto this conceived ovum and enjoy this moment for a while. And this conceived ovum with all its surrounding happy, hormones beautiful chemicals of joy like dopamine, oxytocin and others being bathed in the conceived ovum which has started dividing and the peristalsis takes it forward towards uterus. From 1 it is divided to 2, and 2 into 4 and 4 into 16 and so on and the blastocyst has entered the uterus nearing the fundus of the uterus. Very nice that you have started secreting all the hormones that are required and the blastocyst is settling into the uterus where the endometrium is red, receptive, having very good blood supply and you have succeeded and feeling very very happy, joyful, contented. And now it starts functioning by the nature. From the time immemorial, generation after generations have gone and the same way at the end of 9 months and 10 days, you will have your little one in your hand where you have worked so hard without your knowledge, the nature as made it in such a way that as if without any effort, but on the other hand with all the efforts, it grows to be a healthy foetus and the end of 9 months. Who does this? That question keeps on occurring, but the energy that does not want to reveal in front of us but it keeps on doing naturally. And you are very happy, relaxed and both of you hand in hand just enjoy this situation and when you feel comfortable, you can wake up and have your routine as usual.

My voice is now gradually going away and take your own time to get up and feel fresh and the work that you have started will go on and he will be helping you in all the ways as to whatever you will require. Be peaceful, quiet, happy, joyful and enjoy that you have successfully brought the result that you wanted.

Thank you very much for taking me with you in this journey which was very very pleasant and joyful.

Notes

1. Devotee.
2. Morning prayer.

Index